ELECTRICALLY INFUSED WATER RECIPE BOOK

By

IVANA BARNES

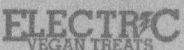

CONTENT

Introduction		3
1.	Lemon Water	5
2.	Lemon Lime Water	7
3.	Lime Mint Water	9
4.	Orange Cinnamon Water	11
5.	Ginger Lime Water	13
6.	Strawberry Lime Water	15
7.	Pineapple Orange Water	17
8.	Blueberry Kiwi Water	19
9.	Lavender Lime Water	21
10.	Strawberry Water	23
11.	Cucumber Mint Water	25
12.	Watermelon Lime Water	27
13.	Watermelon Water	29
14.	Cranberry Lemon Water	31
15.	Pomegranate Water	33
16.	Orange Thyme Water	35
17.	Lemon Lime Orange water	37
18.	Strawberry Cucumber Kiwi Water	39
19.	Cucumber Lemon Lime Water	41
20.	Raspberry Mint Water	43
21.	Blackberry Strawberry Peach Water	45
22.	Orange Kiwi Water	47
23.	Blueberry Lime Water	49
24.	Strawberry Basil Water	51
25.	Watermelon Cucumber Mint Water	53

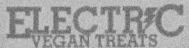

CONTENT

26.	Blueberry Apple Raspberry Water	55
27.	Lemon Thyme Water	57
28.	Cucumber Lime Strawberry Mint Water	59
29.	Orange Star Anise Hibiscus Water	61
30.	Watermelon Honeydew Mint Water	63
31.	Lime Ginger Basil Water	65
32.	Lemon Raspberry Rosemary Water	67
33.	Orange Blueberry Basil Water	69
34.	Ginger Pineapple Apple Water	71
35.	Strawberry Blueberry Water	73
36.	Strawberry Pineapple Water	75
37.	Orange Blueberry Water	77
38.	Apricot Mint Berry Water	79
39.	Peach Plum Mint Water	81
40.	Apple Pear Cinnamon Water	83
41.	Apple Orange Cinnamon Clove Water	85
42.	Grapefruit Rosemary Water	87
43.	Cucumber Thyme Lime Water	89
44.	Cranberry and Orange Water	91
45.	Apple Lime Mint Water	93
46.	Pineapple and Jalapeño Water	95
47.	Blackberry Rosemary Sage Water	97
48.	Cantaloupe Mint Lemon Water	99
49.	Peach and Basil Water	101
50.	Cherry Lime Water	103

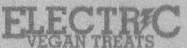

INTRODUCTION

As a registered nurse for over five years, I have learned lack of hydration, healthy foods, electrolytes, vitamins, and minerals are the primary cause of diseases. Most of my patients did not eat healthy or drink a minimum eight glasses of water daily. This was mainly due to lack of resources related to their socioeconomic status. Other patients simply did not have time in their busy schedules to develop healthy eating habits, due to the convenience of fast foods. This is what caused me to begin coaching my patients and ultimately writing this book.

Through coaching patients, this has allowed me to guide them with setting realistic goals. It is my calling to help people take charge of their health while having fun. I created this book to encourage people get more creative with their diet. I truly enjoyed getting innovative with these recipes. These drinks not only taste amazingly delicious, but they are very healthy too. Even your children would love to drink these beverages. I even added a few alcohol recipes in the book too.

By giving people healthier alternatives, I truly believe this will help people stick with their goals so they won't feel so deprived. Completely eliminating certain food items from ones diet can sometimes make it hard for people to stay the course.

To contact us directly, or for more information regarding our company and how we got started, please visit www.electricvegantreats.com. We also can assist with developing a health and wellness program for you, your family, companies, churches, and non-profit organizations.

We would love to keep up with everyone. Please like us at Electric Vegan Treats on Facebook and Instagram as well. Feel free to send us pictures, reviews, and testimonials from our book. We would love to hear from you.

We greatly appreciate your support. Please email us for 10% off on your next purchase. Put in the email message, "10% off code." Thank you so much!

LEMON WATER

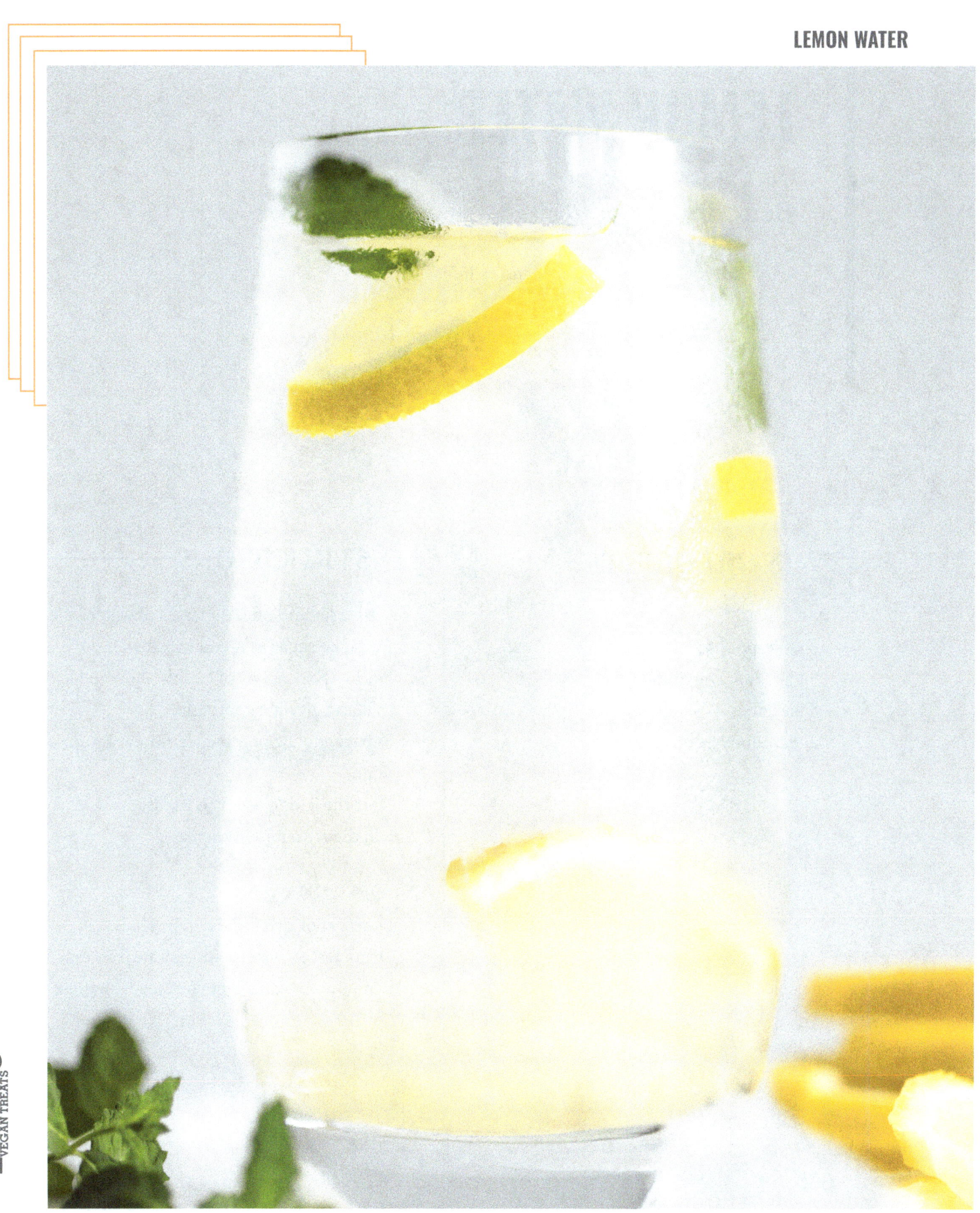

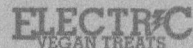

LEMON WATER

Benefits

- Energy boost
- Bloat, constipation, and diarrhea relief
- Detoxing and weight loss
- Cleanse your liver, blood, and kidneys
- Provides vitamin c, magnesium, potassium, and calcium
- Improves the skin
- Decreases bad breath

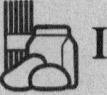

INGREDIENTS

- 6 tablespoons lemon juice
- 3 glasses of cold water
- 6 ice cubes
- 3 teaspoons date sugar

INSTRUCTIONS

1. Grab a jar and pour 3 glasses of water in it.
2. Add date sugar in it and mix it well.
3. Pour 6 tablespoons of freshly squeezed lemon in it and give it a good mix.
4. Refrigerate the prepared lemon water for an hour.
5. Pour the lemon water in 3 glasses and then add the ice cubes in them.

SUGGESTIONS:
1. Don't eat or drink the lemon seeds.
2. Drink lemon water with a straw. Too much lemon water can affect your teeth enamel.

LEMON LIME WATER

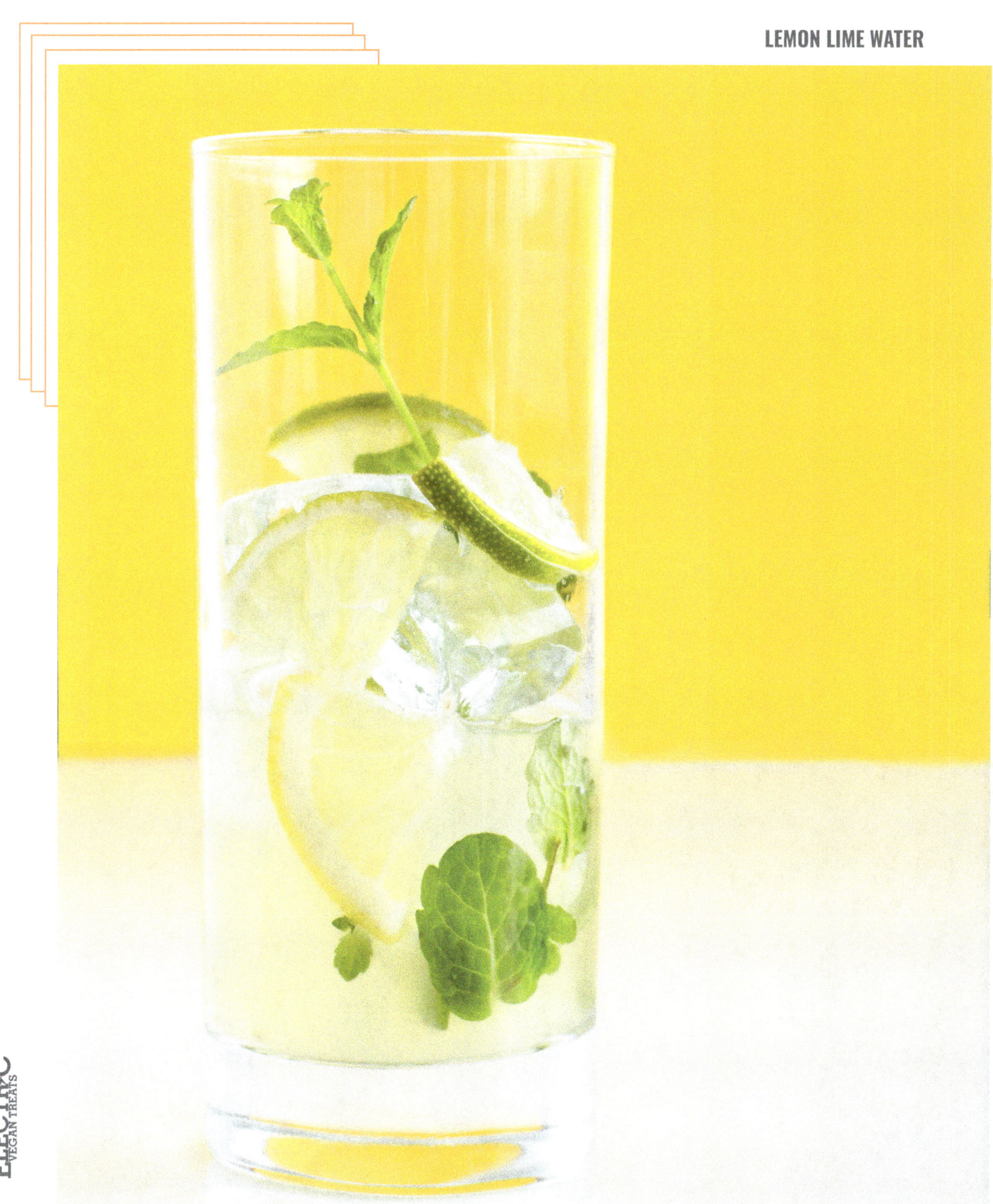

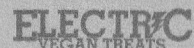

LEMON LIME WATER

Benefits
- Energy boost
- Detox
- Bloat relief
- Vitamin C
- Antiseptic
- Improves skin
- Decreases bad breath
- Helps with weight loss

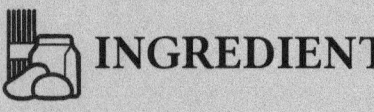 **INGREDIENTS**

- 8 cups of water
- 4 lemons
- 4 lime
- 2 teaspoons agave

 **INSTRUCTIONS**

1. Pour 8 cups of water in a jug.
2. Cut thin slices of lemon and lime and add them in water.
3. Add 2 teaspoons of agave in it and refrigerate it for at least 3 hours.
4. Pour it into the glasses and enjoy it chilled!

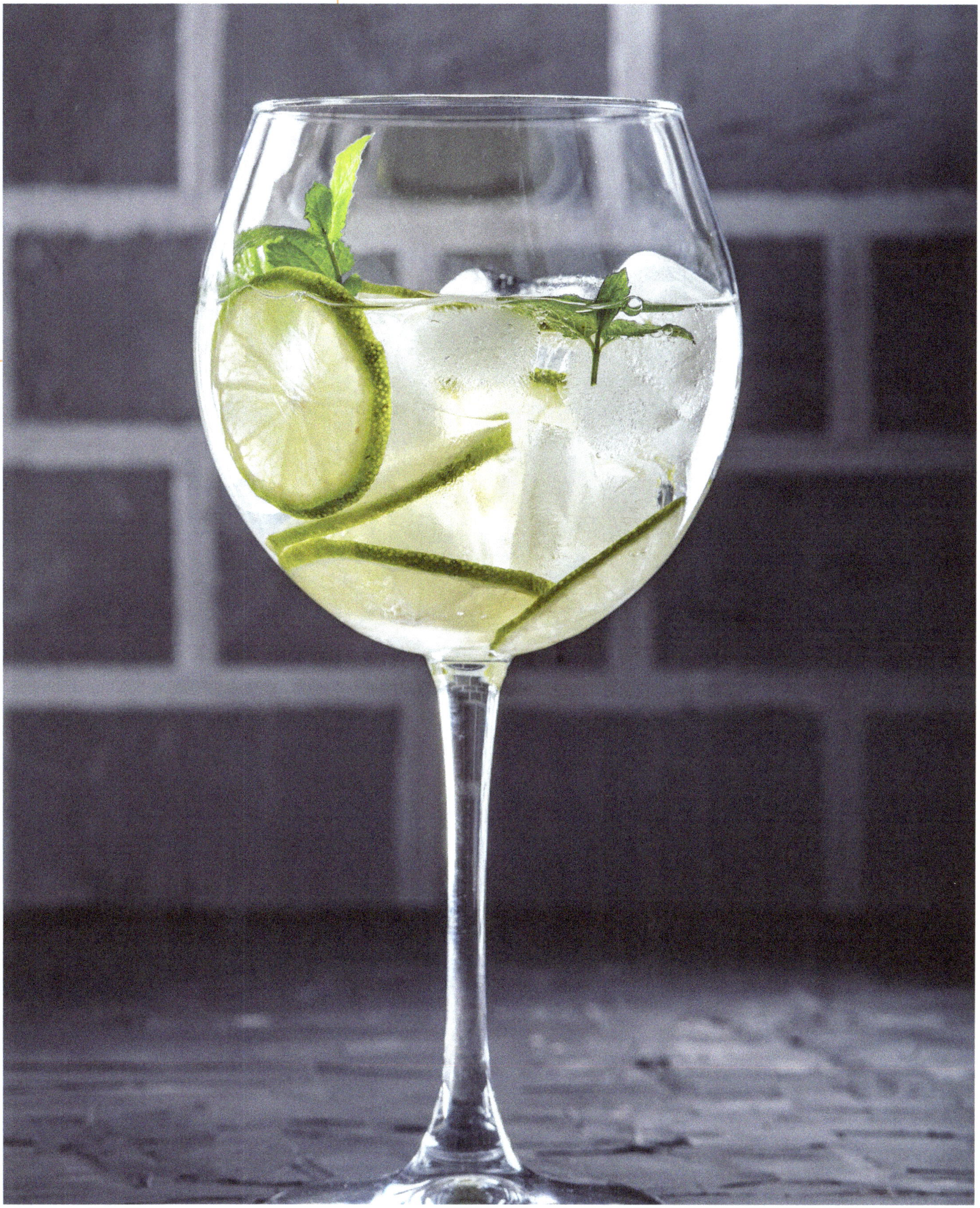

LIME MINT WATER

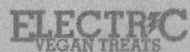

LIME MINT WATER

Benefits
- Skin Improvement
- Helps with Digestion, diarrhea, and irritable bowel syndrome
- Immune system booster
- Helps with weight loss
- Helps regulate blood sugar
- Helps decrease inflammation
- High antioxidants, iron, manganese and vitamin A

 INGREDIENTS

- 4 cups of water
- Juice of 2 limes
- A handful of ice cubes
- 3 sprigs of mint leaves or
- 2 teaspoons agave
- Extra slices of lime

 INSTRUCTIONS

1. Add the slices of lime and sprigs of mint in an empty jug.
2. Grab a blender and pour the lime juice, water and agave into it.
3. Mix them well and prepare a homogenous mixture.
4. Add the ice cubes and pulse it for about 15 seconds.
5. Transfer the prepared juice into the glass and enjoy!

ORANGE CINNAMON WATER

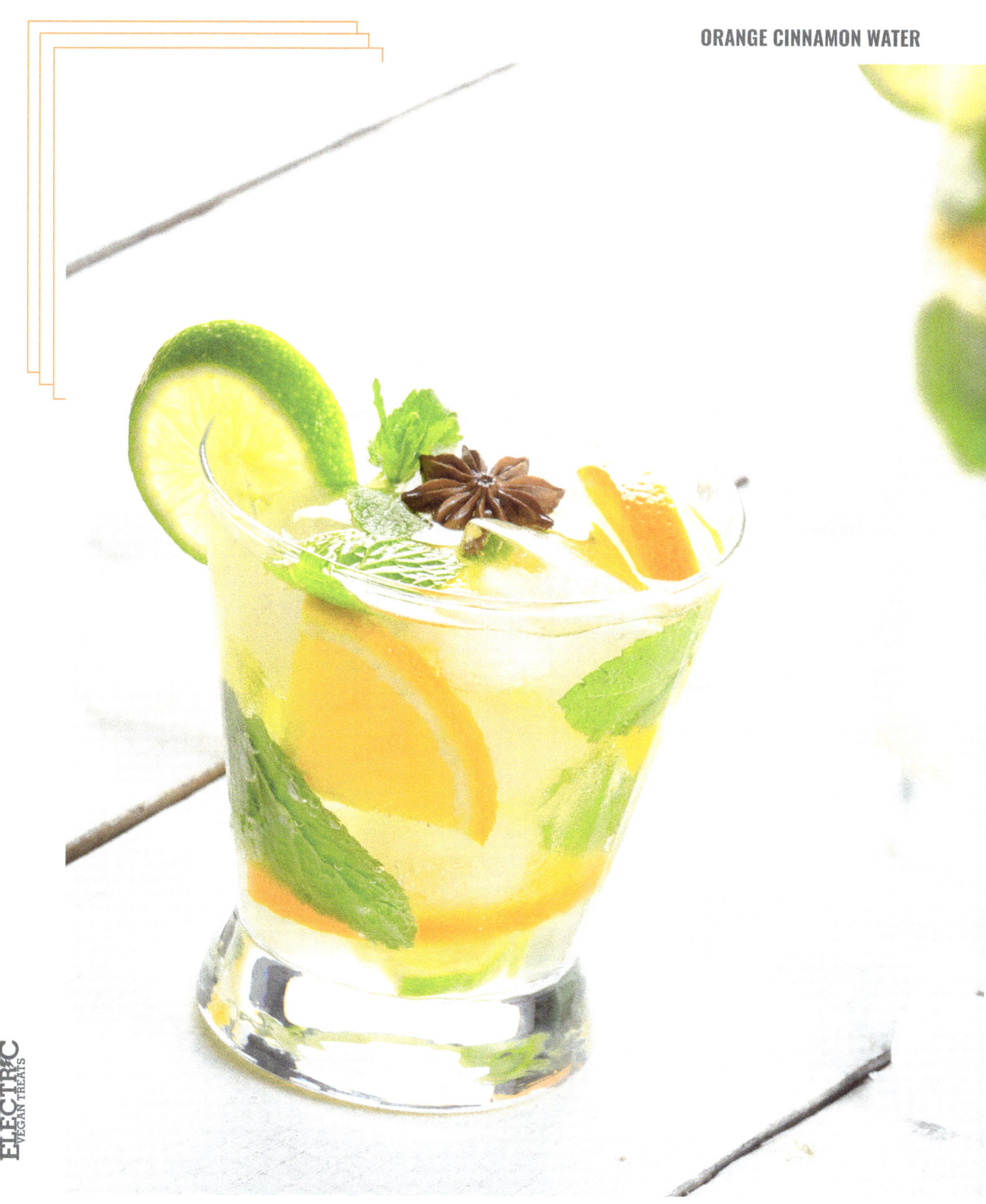

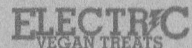

ORANGE CINNAMON WATER

Benefits

- Appetite
- Helps with digestion
- Helps with detox
- Stimulates energy
- Cardiac stimulant
- Soothes sore throat
- Helps lower blood sugar

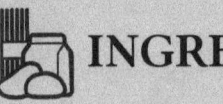 ### INGREDIENTS

 ### INSTRUCTIONS

- 1 teaspoon cinnamon powder
- 1 ounce freshly squeezed orange juice
- 1 glass of sparkling water
- Ice cubes
- Orange slice for garnishing
- 1 cinnamon for garnish

1. Fill ¾ glass with ice cubes.
2. Pour the cinnamon powder and orange juice into the glass.
3. Add the sparkling water over the ice.
4. Stir it to combine well.
5. Garnish with an orange slice and cinnamon and enjoy!

GINGER LIME WATER

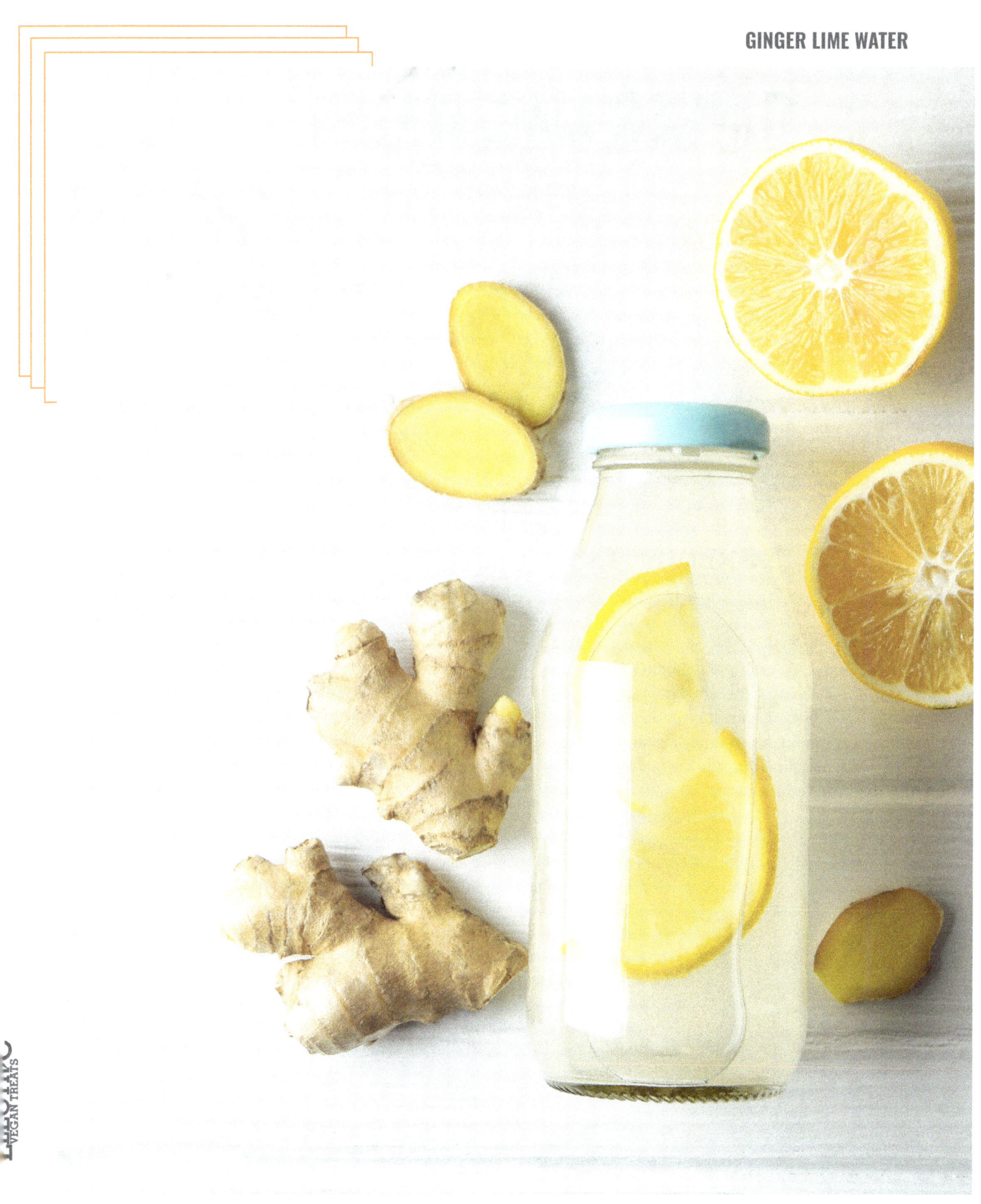

GINGER LIME WATER

Benefits

- Energy boost
- Detoxifying
- Helps with digestion
- Improves your metabolism
- Helps with weight loss
- Relieves heart burn

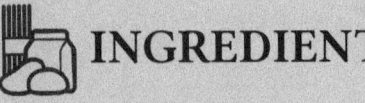 INGREDIENTS

- 2 medium size squeezed lemons
- 1 inch chopped ginger
- ½ cup chilled water
- 500ml sparkling water
- 4-6 tablespoons date sugar
- A pinch of salt

INSTRUCTIONS

1. Grab a blender and add lemon juice, chopped ginger, date sugar, salt into it.
2. Then add the cold water and again blend well for 2-3 minutes.
3. Pulse it over a high speed so that a homogenous mixture is prepared.
4. Pass the mixture through a fine mesh sieve set over a bowl.
5. Discard the remaining solids over the sieve and pour the juice into 2 serving glasses.
6. Add the ice cubes and sparkling water in the end to fill the glass.

STRAWBERRY LIME WATER

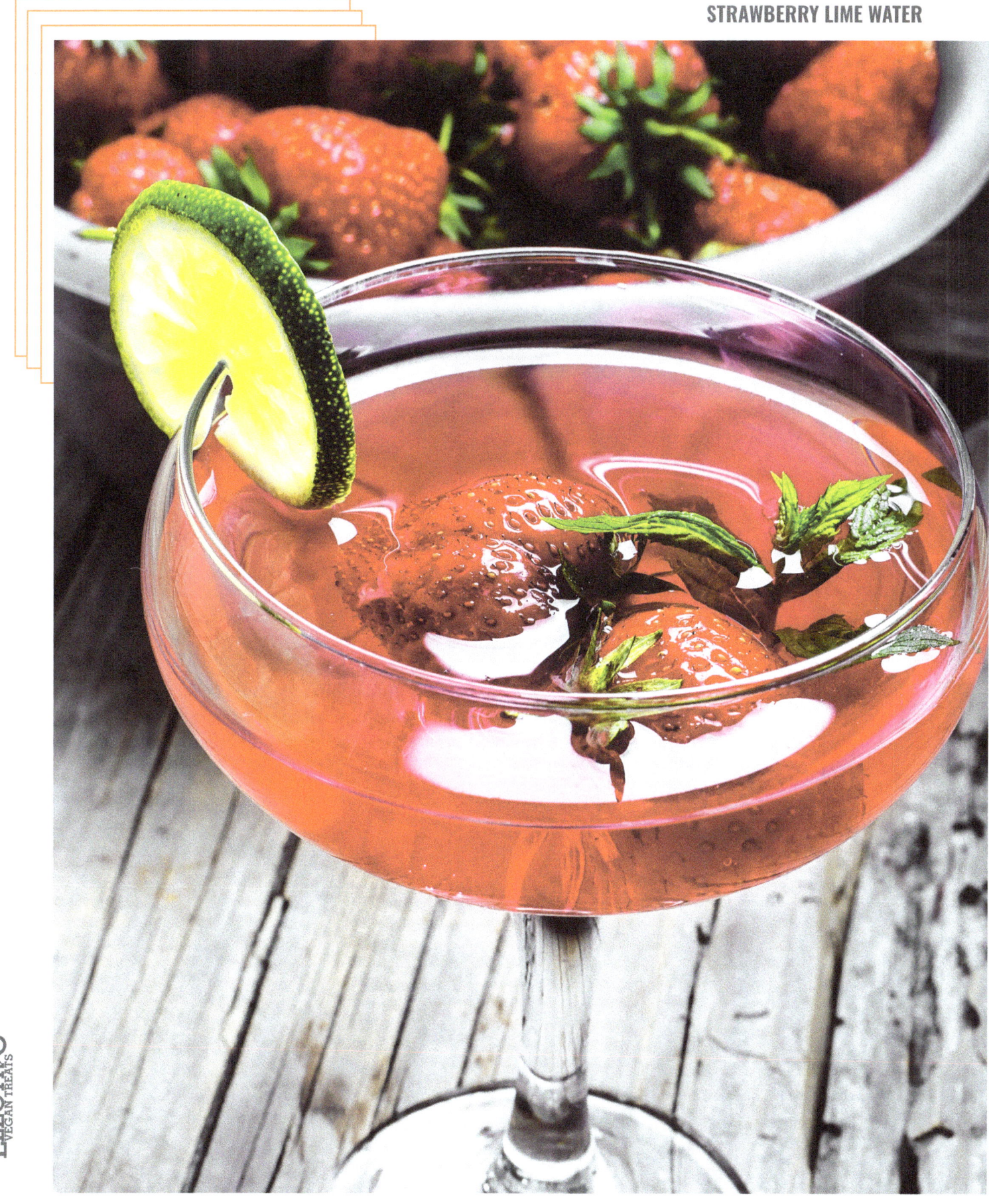

STRAWBERRY LIME WATER

Benefits

- Prevents inflammation
- Boost the immune system
- Helps improve high cholesterol and blood pressure
- Increases urination
- Improves skin
- Prevents constipation
- Helps grow good bacteria
- Great for the nervous system
- Helps prevent cancer

INGREDIENTS

- 1-1/2 cup sliced fresh strawberries
- 1 cup fresh lime juice
- 5 cups of cold water
- 1 cup date sugar
- Ice cubes
- Lime slices for garnishing

INSTRUCTIONS

1. Grab a blender and blend the strawberries and lime juice until smooth.
2. Pour this strawberry and lime mix into a large jug.
3. Add cold water and date sugar.
4. Stir until all the date sugar is dissolved.
5. Pour the prepared juice in the glasses and then add the ice cubes.
6. Garnish with lime, if desired.

PINEAPPLE ORANGE WATER

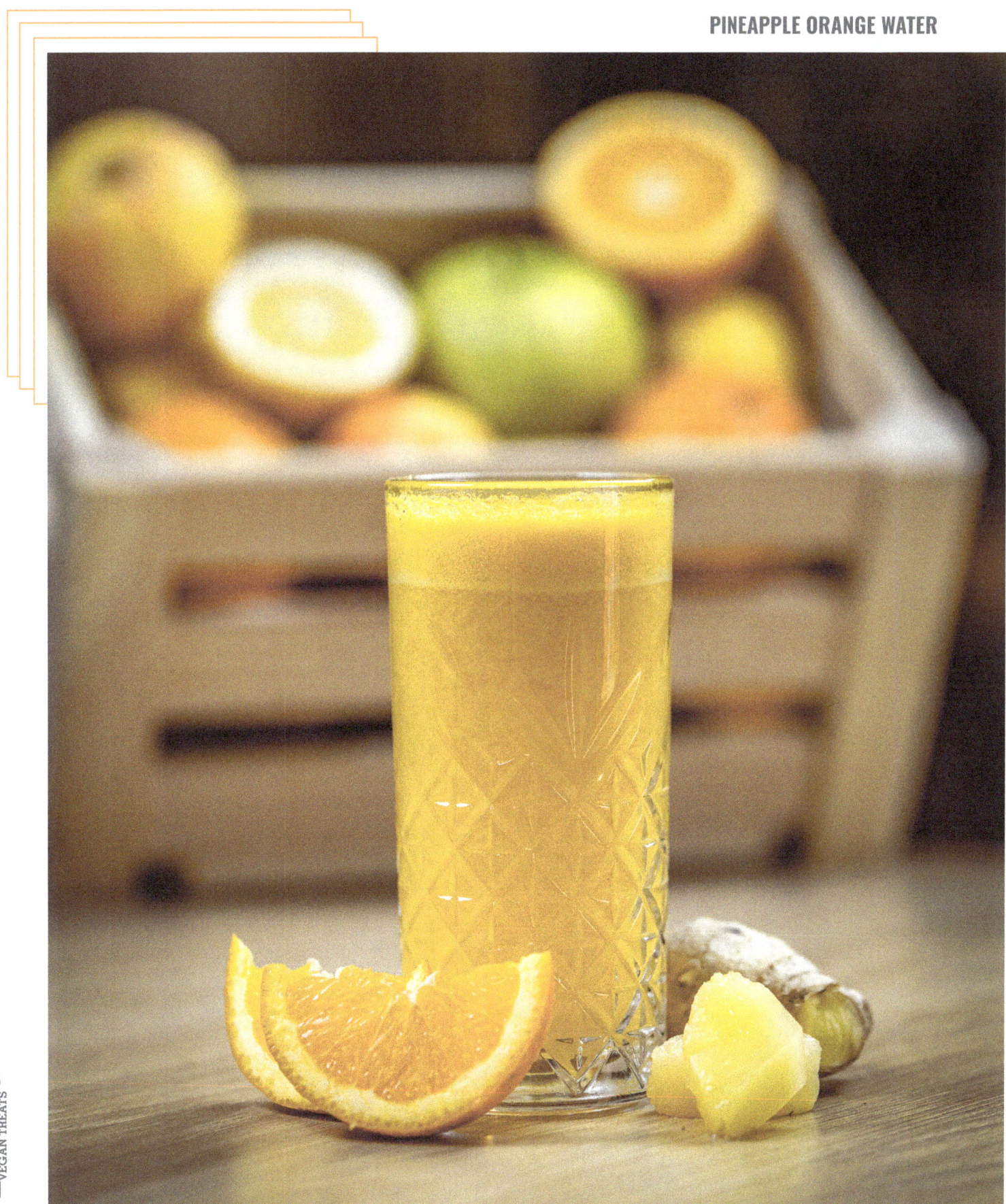

PINEAPPLE ORANGE WATER

Benefits
- High amounts of vitamin A ,B, and C, manganese, and dietary fiber
- Anti-inflammatory

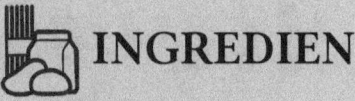 **INGREDIENTS**

- 4 cups water
- ½ cup pineapple chunks
- ½ orange
- 4 tablespoons lime juice

 **INSTRUCTIONS**

1. Pour the water evenly in 4 medium cups.
2. Add equal amount of pineapple chunks, orange slices, agave and one tablespoon of lime juice in each cup.
3. Grab a spoon and mix them well.
4. You may add any sweetener if desired.
5. Chill it in the refrigerator and serve with some ice cubes on the top.

BLUEBERRY KIWI WATER

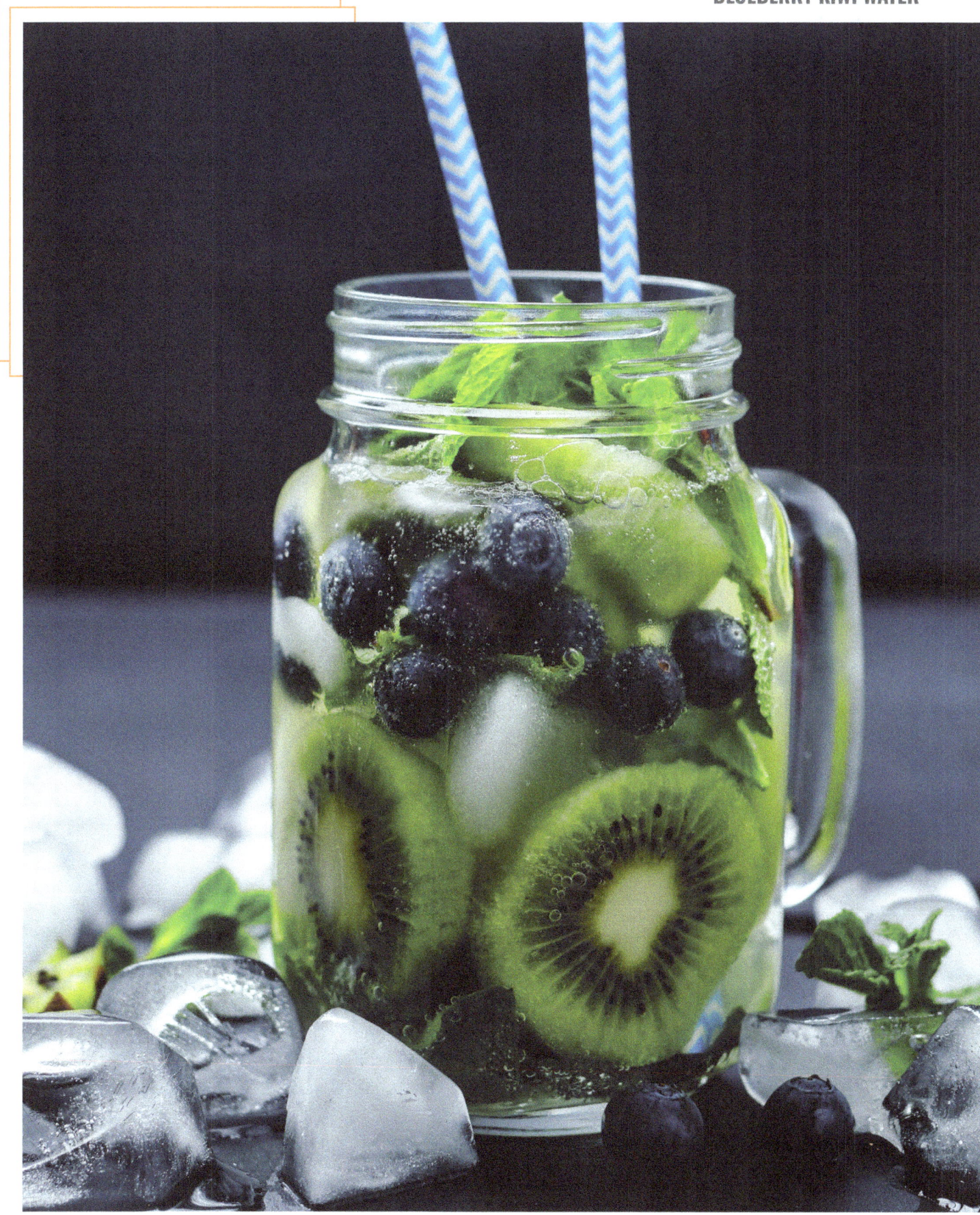

BLUEBERRY KIWI WATER

Benefits
- Keeps skin moisturized
- Promotes healthy hair
- Full of antioxidants and nutrients
- High in vitamin C

INGREDIENTS

FOR THE KIWI LAYER
- 12 peeled and diced kiwis
- 2 tablespoons granulated date sugar
- 1/4 cup water

FOR THE BLUEBERRIES LAYER
- 2 cups frozen blueberries
- 1 tablespoon granulated date sugar
- 2 tablespoons water

INSTRUCTIONS

FOR THE KIWI LAYER
1. Grab a blender and add kiwi slices in it.
2. Blend them well to make a thick puree.
3. Now add date sugar and ¼ cup water.
4. Again give it a good mix so that the date sugar is combined well.
5. Check the consistency of the mixture by adding a teaspoon of water one by one.
6. Now divide this mixture between 4 glasses and fill them half way up.

FOR THE BLUEBERRIES LAYER

7. In a blender, combine all the ingredients and pulse them at high speed until a smooth mixture forms.
8. More water can be added to reach desired consistency.
9. Pour it over the kiwi filling in the glasses all the way up.
10. Serve it chilled for at least 2 hours.

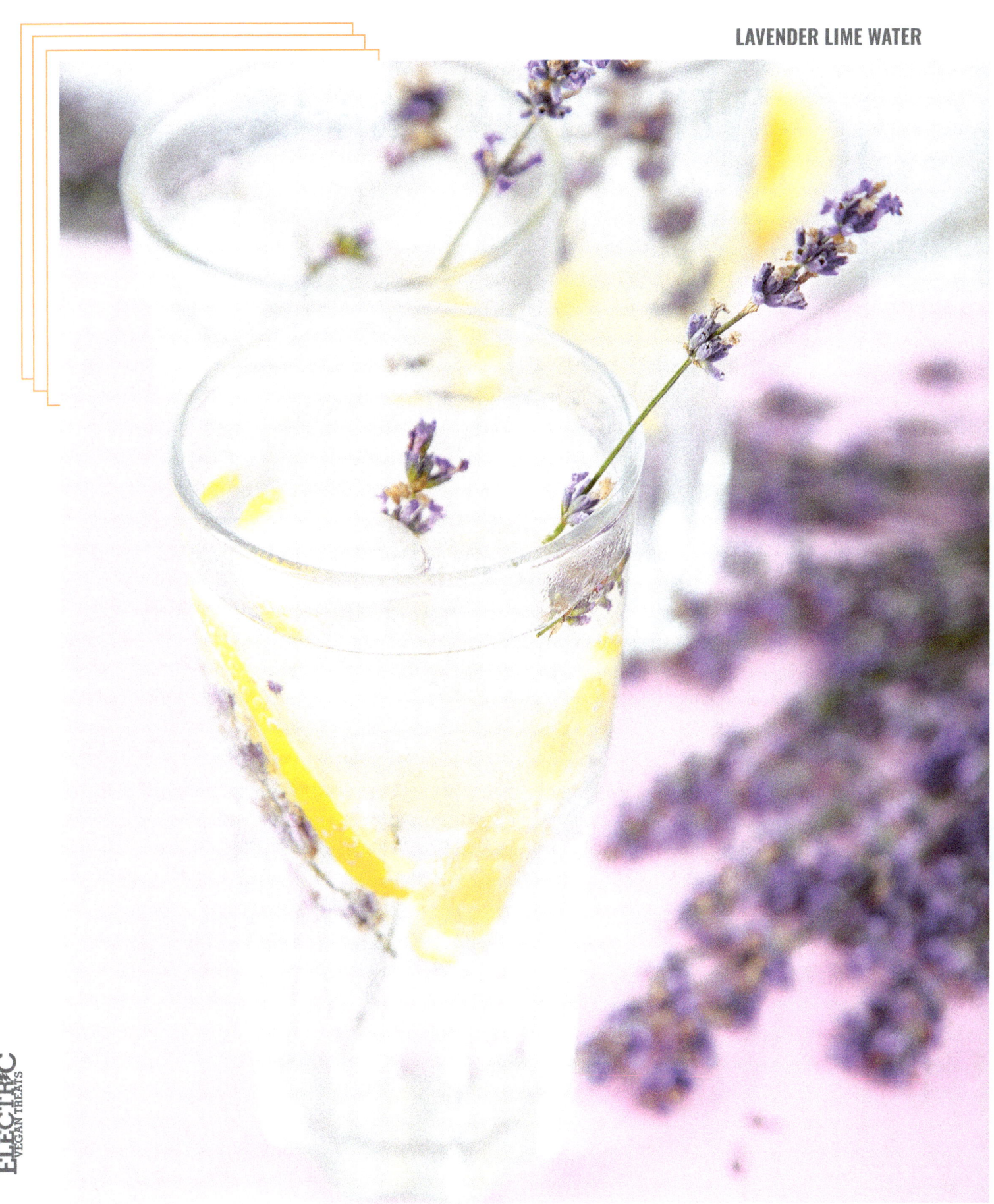

LAVENDER LIME WATER

LAVENDER LIME WATER

Benefits
- Calming affect
- Improves mood disorders like depression, anxiety, and fatigue
- Used as an aromatherapy agent
- Boost sleep
- Helps soothe menstrual cramping
- Helps improve skin
- Boosts Immune system
- Reduces inflammation

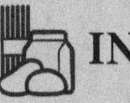 ## INGREDIENTS

FOR THE LAVENDER SIMPLE SYRUP
- 2 cups of cold water
- 2 cups date sugar
- 1/4 cup dried lavender flowers

FOR THE LAVENDER-LIME SODA
- 1/3 cup Lavender Simple Syrup
- 1/4 cup freshly squeezed lime juice
- 1 cup sparkling water

 ## INSTRUCTIONS

MAKE THE SIMPLE SYRUP
1. Grab a saucepan and add water, date sugar, and lavender in it.
2. Bring it to boil until all of the date sugar is dissolved.
3. Remove from heat and then allow to cool down for at least half an hour.
4. Take a sieve and then strain the mixture into a jar.
5. Now refrigerate it before using.

MAKE THE LAVENDER-LIME SODA
6. Add the lavender simple syrup and lime juice together in medium jar.
7. Pour the club soda over it.
8. Enjoy!

STRAWBERRY WATER

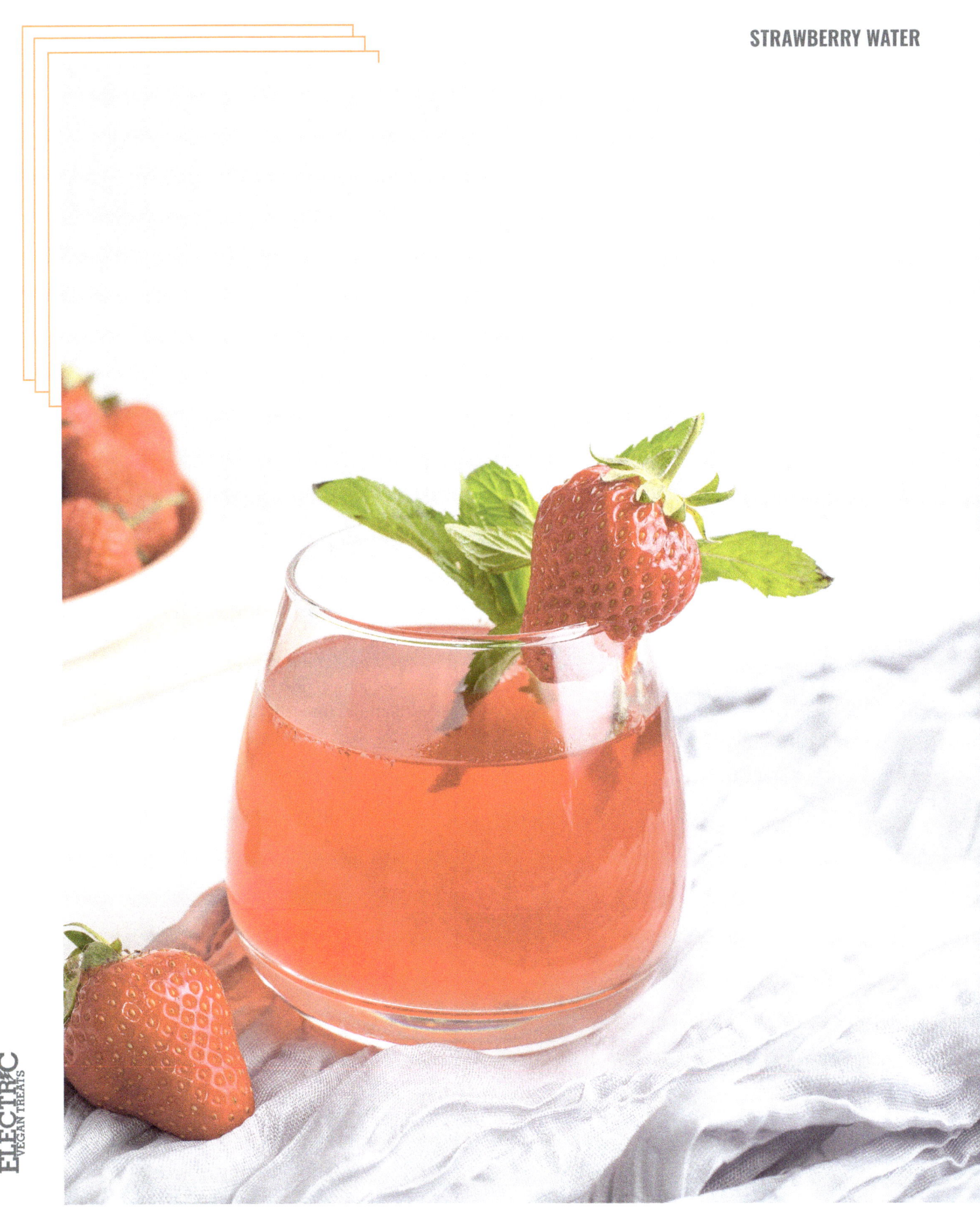

STRAWBERRY WATER

Benefits
- Flush out toxins
- Helps improve skin tone
- Keeps you hydrated
- High levels of antioxidants called polyphenols
- Vitamin C

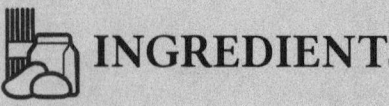 INGREDIENTS

- 2 cups Strawberries
- 1 teaspoon Lemon juice
- 2 tablespoon Date sugar
- A pinch of Salt
- 2 cups Chilled Water
- Ice cubes

 INSTRUCTIONS

1. Rinse the strawberries, tap them to dry and then roughly chop them into slices.
2. Grab a blender and add chopped strawberries, lemon juice, date sugar and salt.
3. Blend them well till you get smooth puree of strawberries.
4. Add chilled water and blend for a few seconds.
5. Use a strainer if you do not want any crunch. (optional)
6. Pour into serving glasses and add the ice cubes.

CUCUMBER MINT WATER

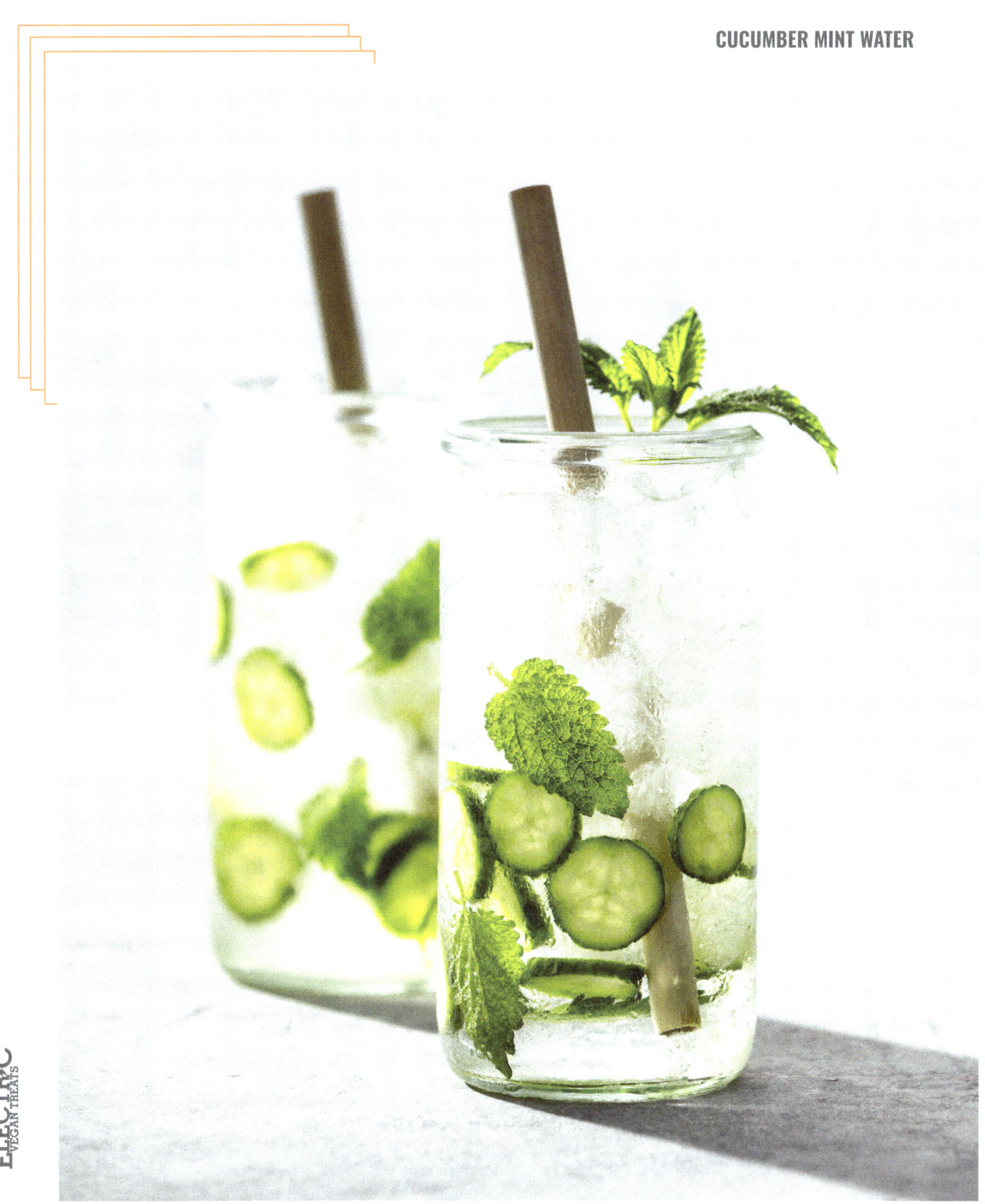

CUCUMBER MINT WATER

Benefits
- Keeps you hydrated
- Aids in weight loss
- High in antioxidants
- Helps lower blood pressure
- Supports healthy skin
- Aids in bone health

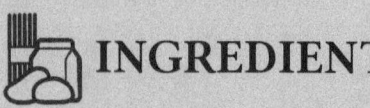 

INGREDIENTS

- 1 medium-size cucumber stripped and cut into 3D squares
- 10-12 mint leaves
- 3 tbsp. date sugar syrup
- 3 tbsp. lemon juice
- ½ tsp salt
- ¼ tsp pink salt
- 3 cup water or as required
- Ice cubes

INSTRUCTIONS

1. Take a blender and add cleaved cucumber.
2. Then, at that point add mint leaves and 1 cup water. Mix it well until smooth.
3. Spot a fine-network sifter or a cheesecloth over an enormous blow away to strain the juice.
4. Strain it and utilize the spoon to press the solids to take out all the juice. There will be around 1-1/4 cups of cucumber juice.
5. Dispose of the mash. After this, add date sugar syrup, and pink salt, and lemon juice.
6. Blend it well. Add the leftover water to the cucumber juice.
7. Pour the cucumber juice into the glass. Put some ice cubes.

WATERMELON LIME WATER

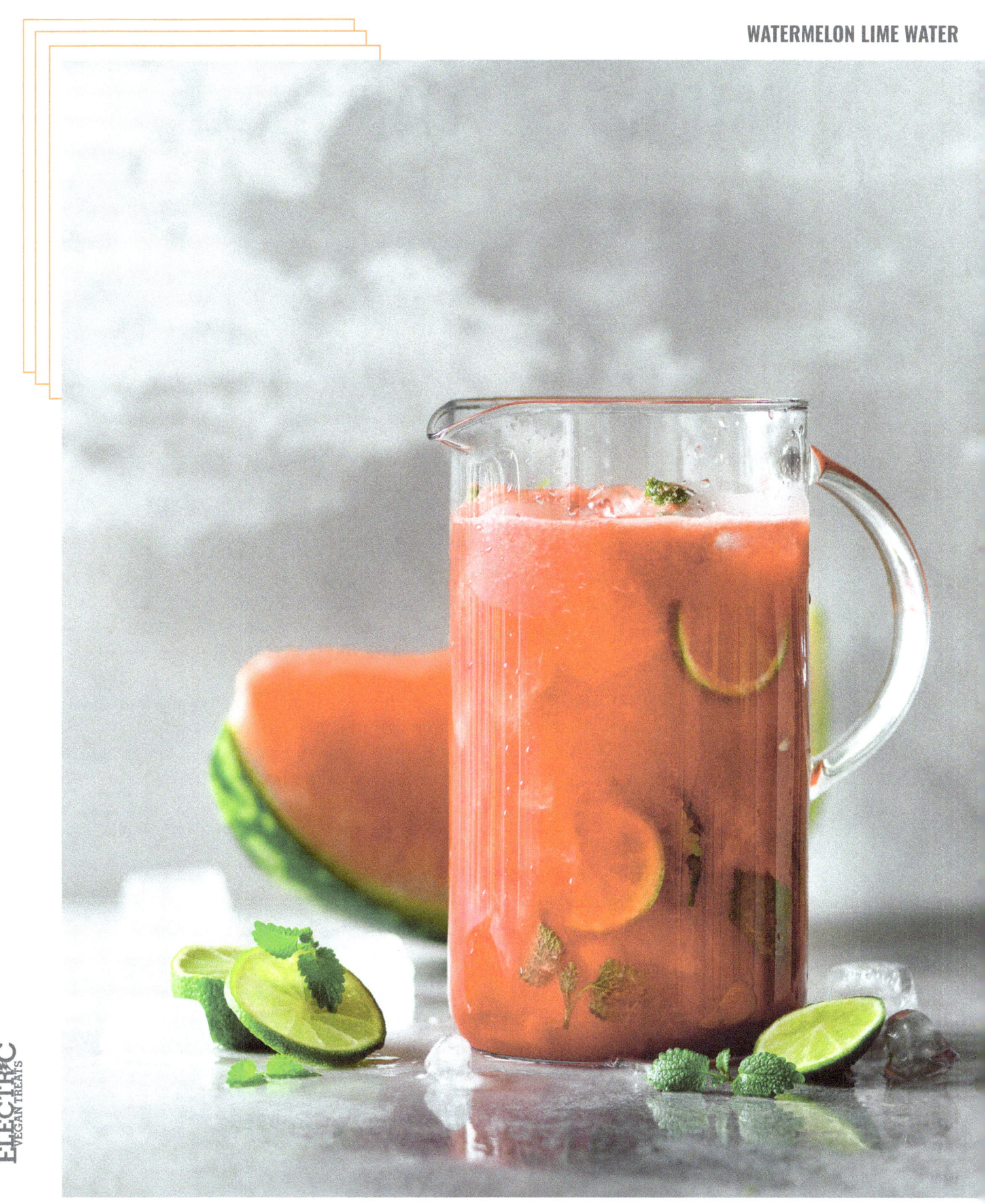

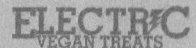

WATERMELON LIME WATER

Benefits
- Detoxifying
- Great for weight loss
- Boosts immune system
- Improves liver function
- High in vitamin c
- Good source of potassium, vitamin A,B,C,D, calcium, and magnesium

 INGREDIENTS

- ¾ cup date sugar
- ½ cup water
- ¼ cup cleaved stripped new ginger
- 10 cups diced watermelon
- ¾ cup new lime juice
- 4 cups chilled soda
- Ice cubes

 INSTRUCTIONS

1. Consolidate sugar, water, and ginger in a little pan over high warmth.
2. Cook until sugar dissolves, mixing with a whisk.
3. Eliminate from heat; cover and let stand 15 minutes. Strain; dispose of solids.
4. Add water-sugar mix, diced watermelon and lime juice in a jug.
5. Let it infuse for 3 hours.
6. Pour sparkling water in the jug and add some ice cubes.

WATERMELON WATER

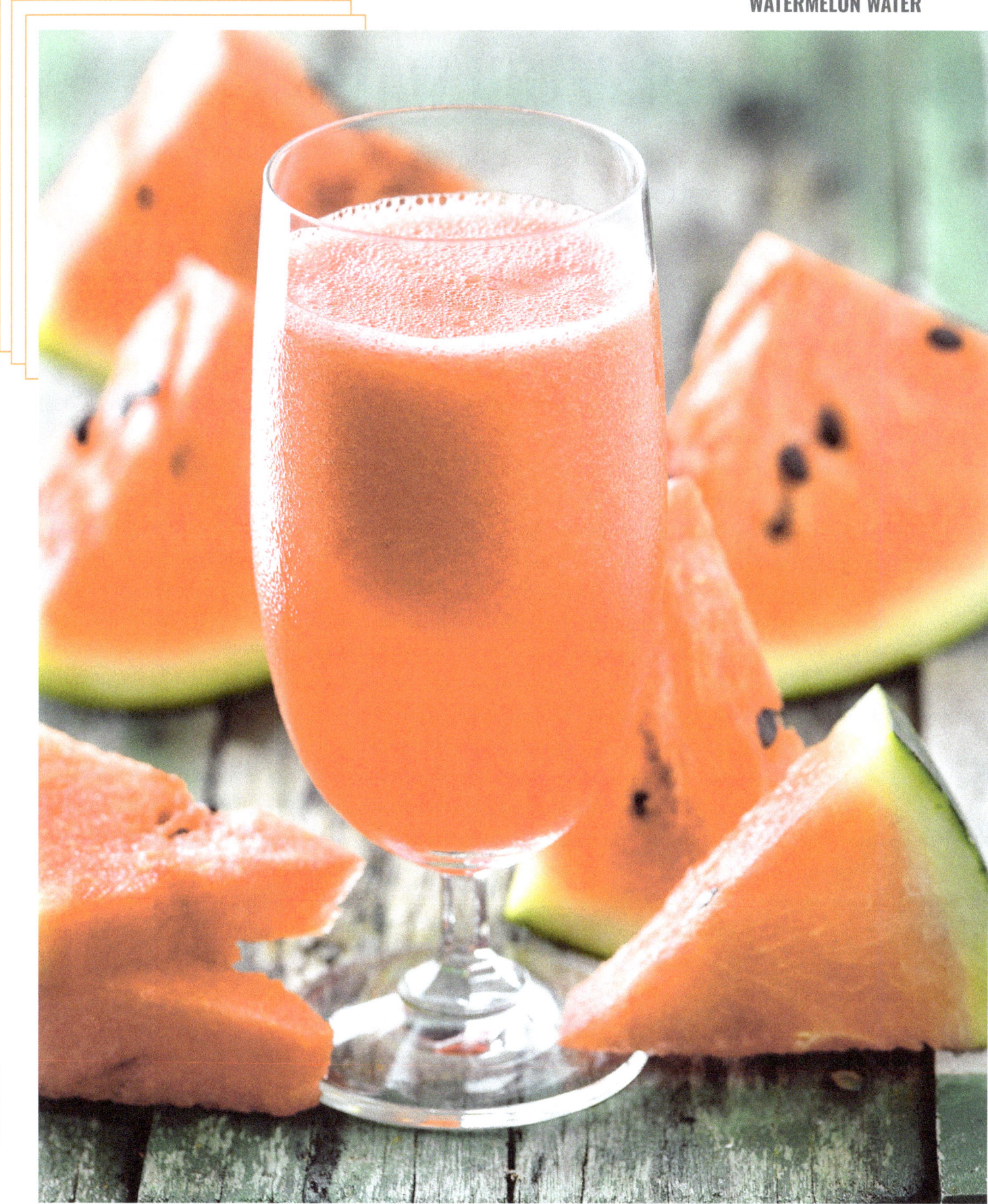

WATERMELON WATER

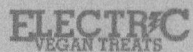

Benefits
- High in vitamin A,B, C, and potassium
- Full of antioxidants
- Anti-inflammatories
- Hydrating

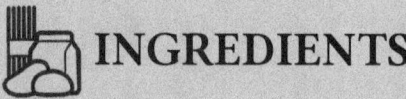 INGREDIENTS

- 1 little sweet watermelon
- 4 cups water

 INSTRUCTIONS

1. Cut the watermelon down the middle.
2. Utilizing a major spoon, scoop pieces of sweet watermelon into the blender.
3. Dispose of the skin.
4. Mix the watermelon until it is completely crushed. This shouldn't take over a moment.
5. In the event that your watermelon is prominently thick or cultivated, pour the blend through a fine cross-section sifter into a jug.
6. If not, you can empty it into glasses loaded up with ice.
7. Watermelon juice can be kept in the fridge, covered, for as long as 4 days.
8. The juice will isolate after some time; mix it with a spoon to recombine.

CRANBERRY LEMON WATER

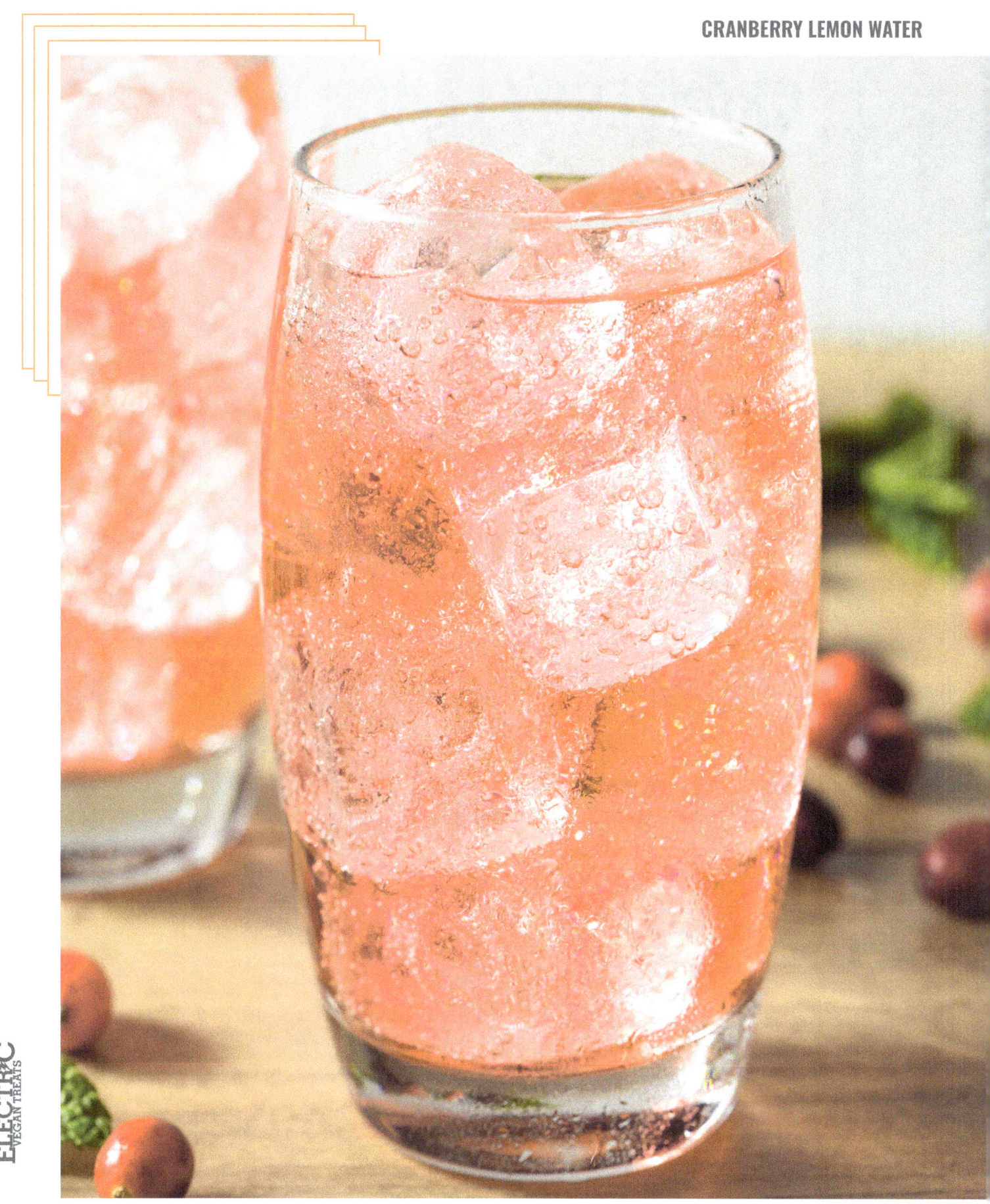

CRANBERRY LEMON WATER

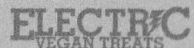

Benefits
- Lowers risk of UTIs
- Improved immune function
- Helps decrease blood pressure
- Helps treat poor appetite
- Aids in weight loss and reduces inflammation
- Full of vitamin A, B,C, E, K, potassium phosphorus, calcium, iron, and fiber

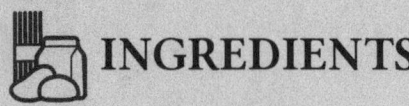

 INSTRUCTIONS

Ingredients
- 3/4 cup date sugar
- 2/3 cup lemon juice
- 3 cups cold water
- 1 cup fresh cranberry

Instructions
1. In a small saucepan, combine date sugar and lemon juice.
2. Cook and stir over medium heat until date sugar is dissolved.
3. Stir in the water and fresh cranberry.
4. If you don't have access then you may also use real cranberry juice.
5. Refrigerate until chilled.
6. Serve over with ice.

POMEGRANATE WATER

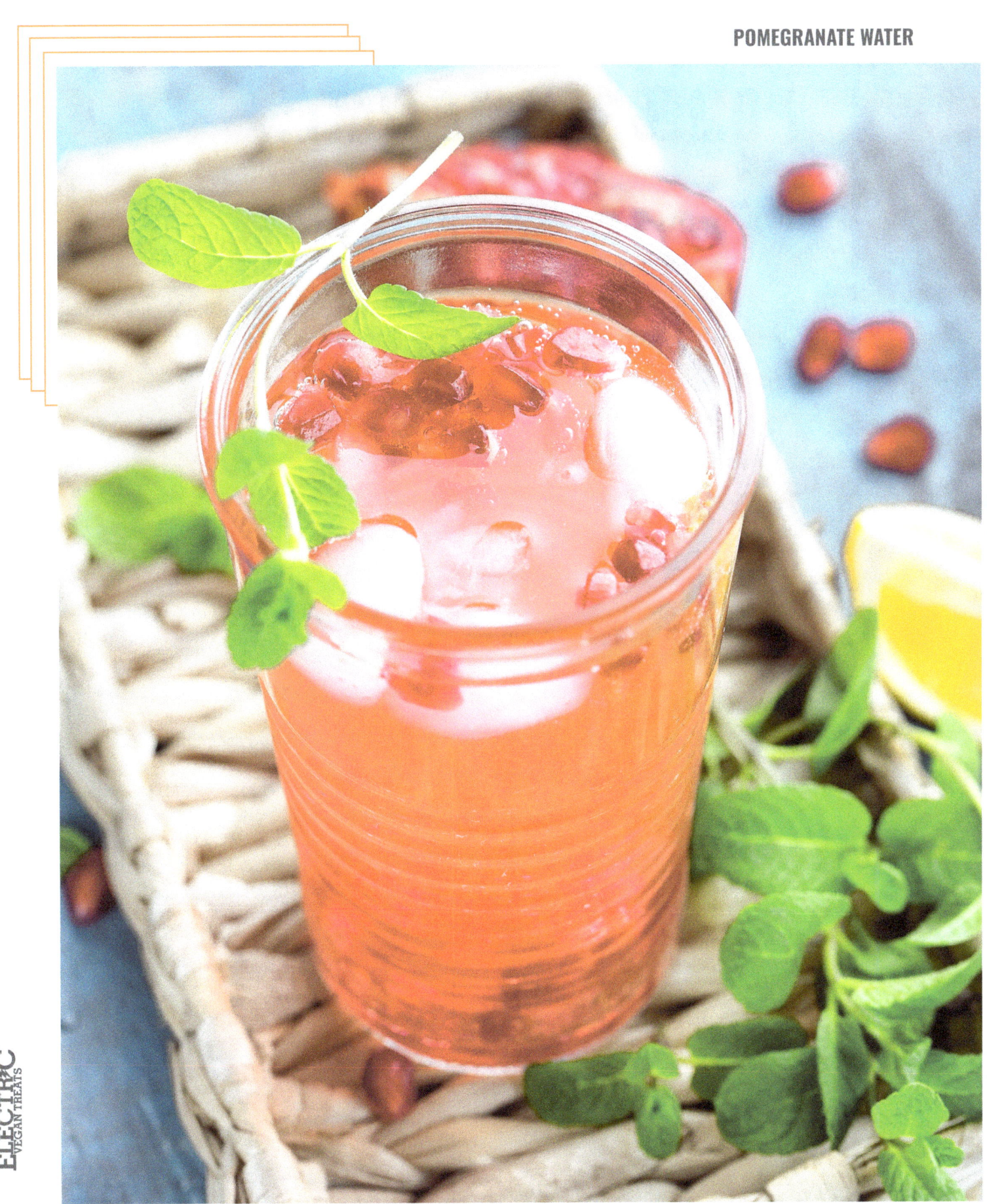

POMEGRANATE WATER

Benefits

- Full of Antioxidants
- Vitamin C
- Great for brain health
- Aids in digestion
- Anti-inflammatory
- Assists with arthritis
- Antiviral Properties
- Full of vitamin C,E,K, folate and potassium
- Helps improve memory
- Helps improve sexual performance and fertility
- Aids with endurance and sports performance
- Helps with managing diabetes

INGREDIENTS

- 1 pomegranate
- 5 cm ginger
- Limes, 1 medium

INSTRUCTIONS

1. Cut off the top of the pomegranate.
2. Cut through the shell at the segments and break the fruit open.
3. Remove the seeds and place them in a large jug.
4. Peel the ginger and slice thinly. Thinly slice the lime.
5. Add to the pomegranate seeds in the jug.
6. Fill the jug with water and serve with ice cubes or leave in the fridge for a few hours.
7. The longer the water is left to stand, the more the flavor will develop.

ORANGE THYME WATER

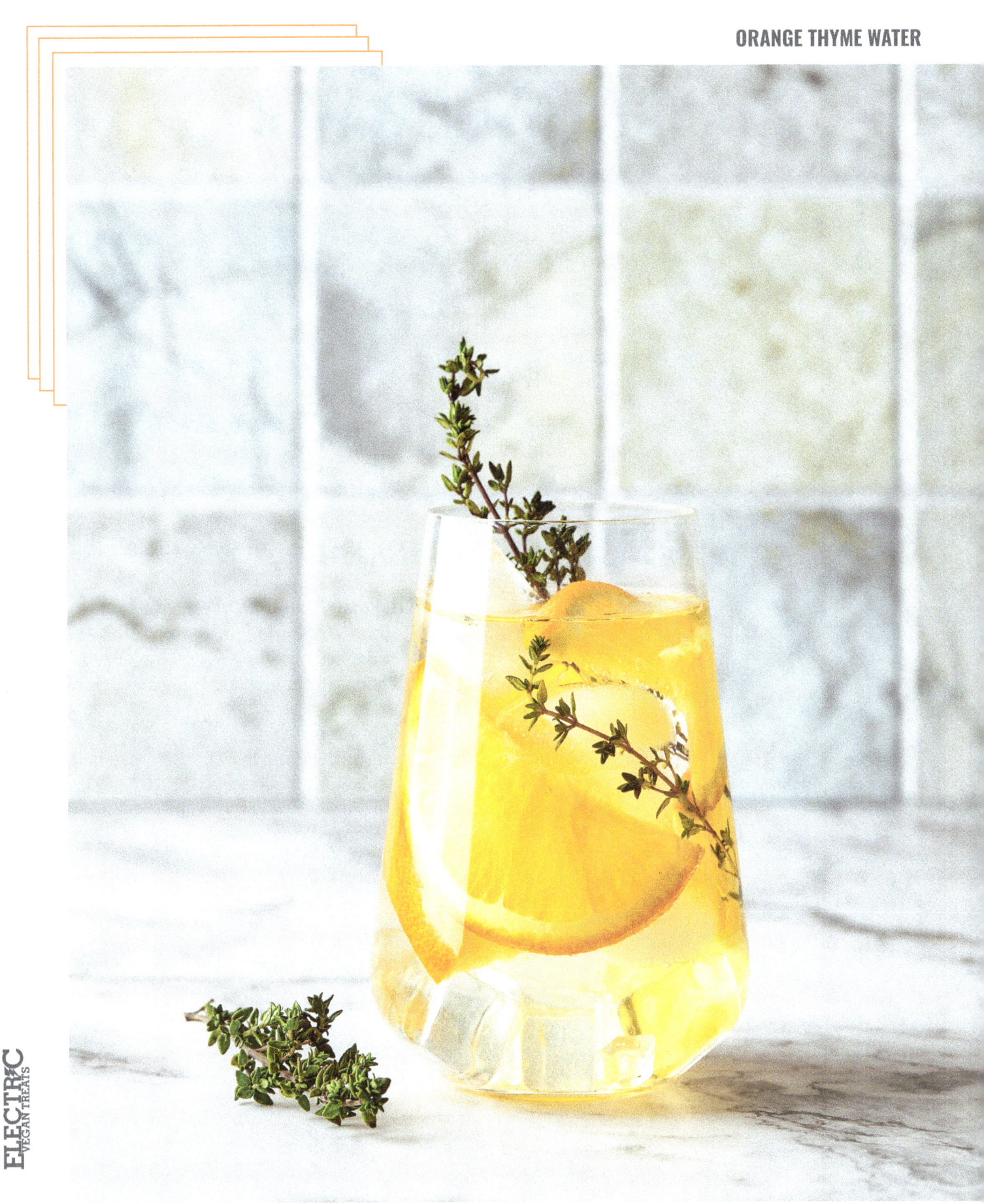

ORANGE THYME WATER

Benefits
- Helps stimulates metabolism
- Helps improve mood
- Diuretic
- Detoxification
- Assists with weight loss
- Assist with dispelling yeast

INGREDIENTS

- 2 cups freshly squeezed orange/real orange juice
- 2 cups Champagne

AGAVE THYME SYRUP:
- 1/2 cup water
- 1/2 cup crude agave
- 6 3-inch twigs new thyme

INSTRUCTIONS

1. Add water, agave, and thyme in a saucepan.
2. Bring to a stew until the agave has consolidated completely.
3. Eliminate from heat and let thyme steep for 30 minutes.
4. Strain out thyme.
5. Transfer the syrup to a jar and keep it in the refrigerator.
6. Pour 2 oz. of thyme syrup into every one of four mixed drink glasses.
7. Add ½ cup champagne and squeezed orange to each glass. Serve.

LEMON LIME ORANGE WATER

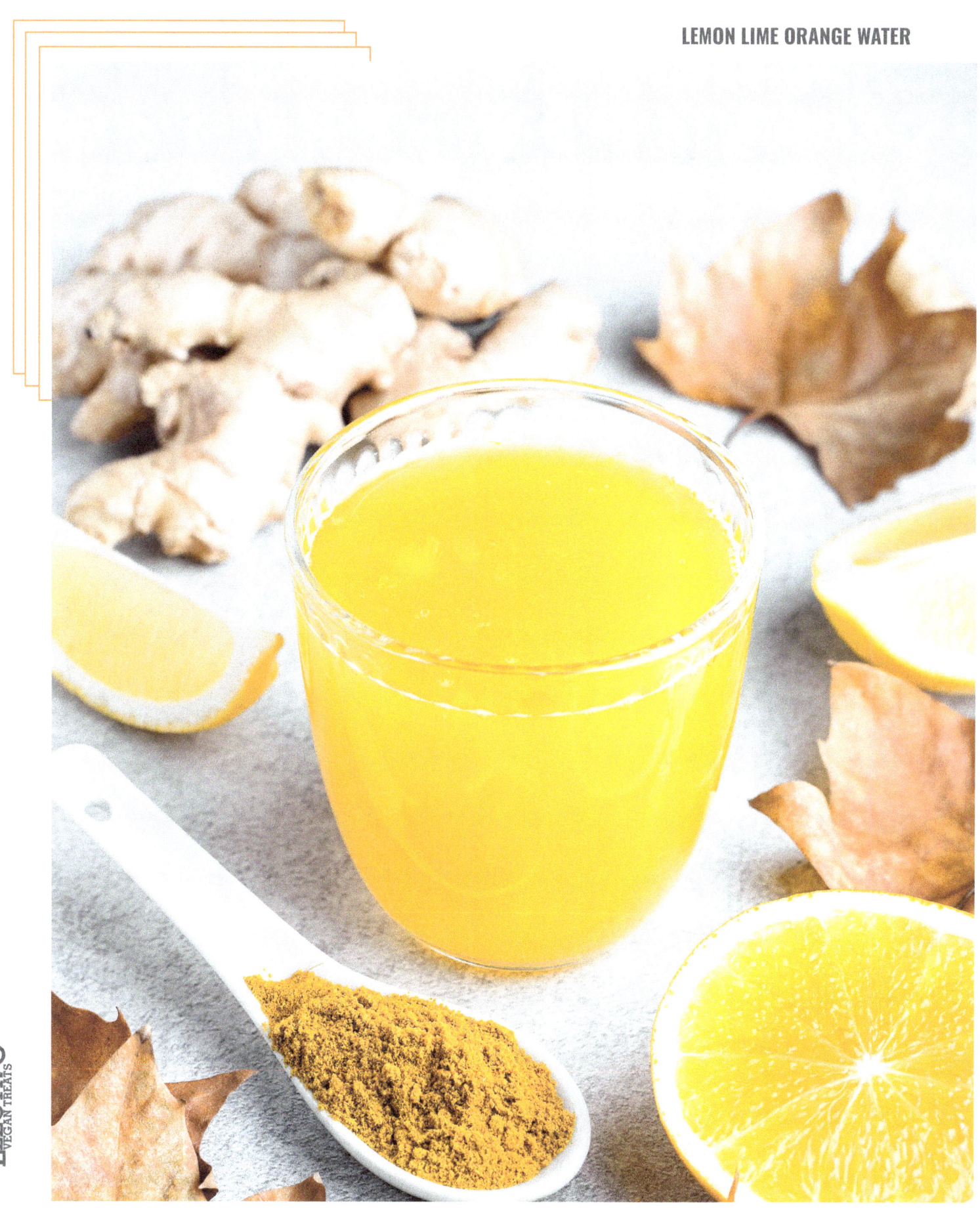

LEMON LIME ORANGE WATER

Benefits
- Good source of vitamin C
- Alkalizing properties
- High in vitamin A and C, calcium, potassium, and pectin

INGREDIENTS

- 1 medium orange
- ½ medium lemon
- ½ medium lime
- 1 medium grapefruit, stripped
- (1-inch) piece fresh ginger root, stripped
- (1-inch) piece fresh turmeric root, stripped
- ½ clove garlic
- A pinch of fresh ground dark pepper

INSTRUCTIONS

1. In a jug, combine grapefruit, juice from the orange.
2. Also add lime, lemon, ginger, turmeric and garlic.
3. Mix the ingredients with a spoon.
4. Spot a little sifter or sifter over a jar container or glass cup.
5. Empty fluid into a sifter and serve promptly
6. Store in the fridge for as long as 4 days.

STRAWBERRY CUCUMBER KIWI WATER

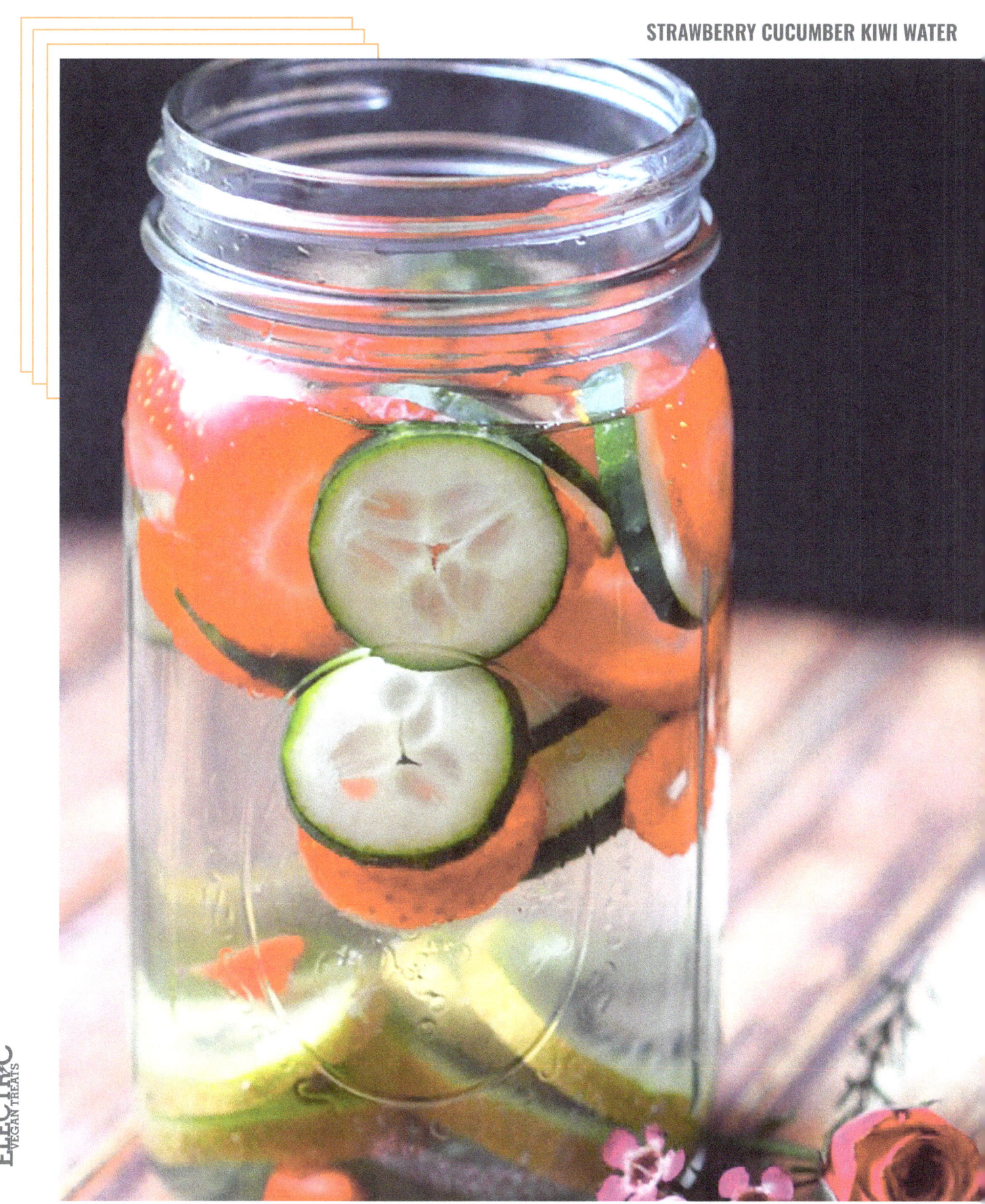

STRAWBERRY CUCUMBER KIWI WATER

Benefits

- Helps improve diabetes
- Weight loss
- Hydration
- Boosts metabolism
- Boosts immune system
- Appetite control
- Detoxifying

INGREDIENTS

- 6 fresh strawberries, hulled
- 1 enormous cucumber, stripped and cut into lumps
- 1 medium kiwi
- 1 huge red apple, cut into eighths
- Ice (discretionary)

INSTRUCTIONS

1. Grab a jug and add strawberries, cucumbers, kiwi and apples to it.
2. Let them infuse for 3 hours.
3. Fill 2 glasses with ice and transfer the infused water into the glasses.
4. Serve right away.

CUCUMBER LEMON LIME WATER

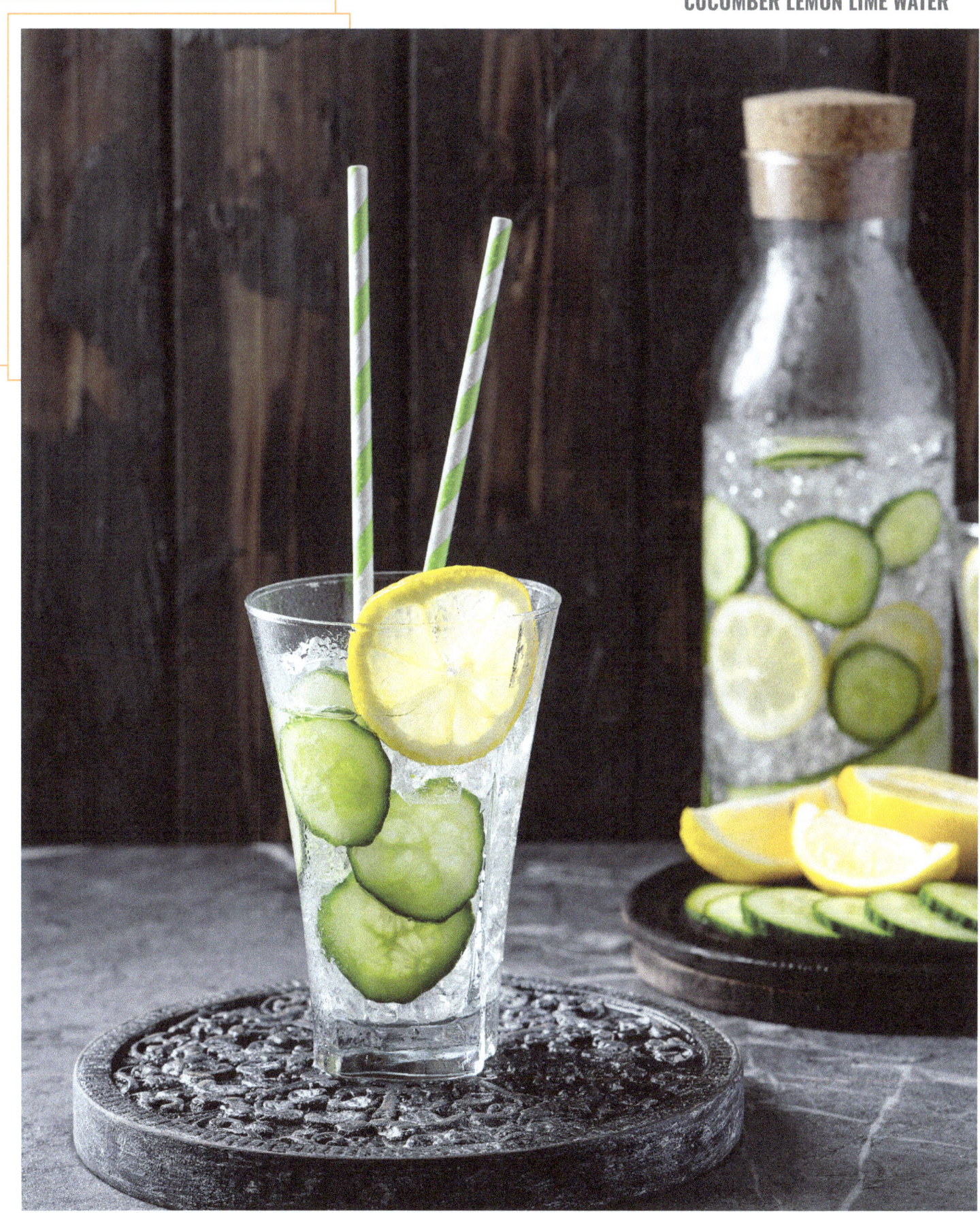

CUCUMBER LEMON LIME WATER

Benefits

- Helps maintain body fluids
- Kidney detox
- Improves skin
- Lowers blood pressure
- Helps fight infections
- Reduces bloating
- Appetite control

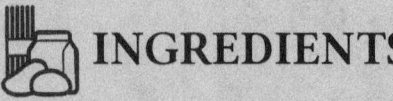 INGREDIENTS

- 6 cups water
- 2 medium cucumbers
- 1 lemon squeeze
- 1 lime zest
- 2 tablespoons fresh mint

 INSTRUCTIONS

1. Cut off the closures of the cucumbers and strip. Slash into a couple of bigger parts.
2. Spot the cucumbers, water, lemon zing, lemon squeeze, and mint in a food processor or a blender.
3. Mix the elements for 2-3 minutes until smooth.
4. Set a sifter over a bigger bowl and empty the cucumber juice into the sifter.
5. Utilize a spatula to move the juice through the sifter until no more squeeze strains out.
6. Dispose of the extra solids.
7. Pour it into the jar and then drink the cucumber squeeze quickly.
8. Or store in the refrigerator for as long as 24 hours.

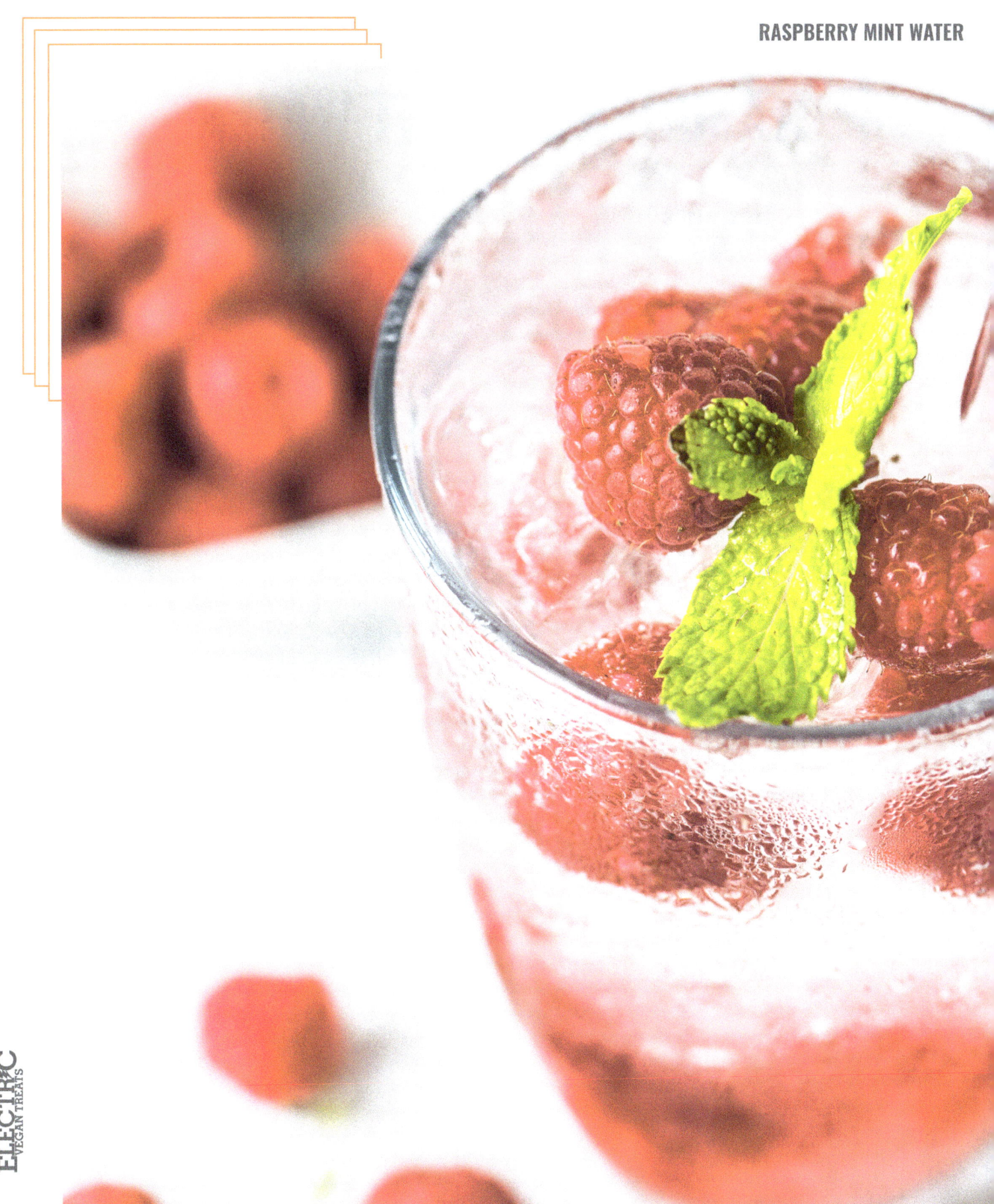

RASPBERRY MINT WATER

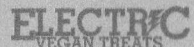

RASPBERRY MINT WATER

Benefits

- High in vitamin C
- Improves memory
- Lowers the risk of obesity and heart disease
- Improves digestion
- Detoxifying
- Increases energy

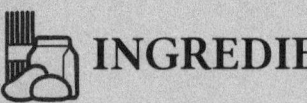 

INGREDIENTS

- 1/3 cup fresh raspberries
- 2 limes, each cut into 4 wedges
- 4 tablespoons date sugar
- 12-16 fresh mint leaves
- 4 oz. white rum
- 8-10 oz. soda
- Ice for serving

INSTRUCTIONS

1. Add the lime wedges, date sugar, mint leaves, raspberries, and rum between two glasses.
2. Utilizing a muddler or the rear of a wooden spoon, crush fixings for 1-2 minutes or until juices start to deliver.
3. Add a couple of ice solid shapes to each glass.
4. Top each with 4-8 oz. club soda.
5. Serve promptly and relish!

BLACKBERRY STRAWBERRY PEACH WATER

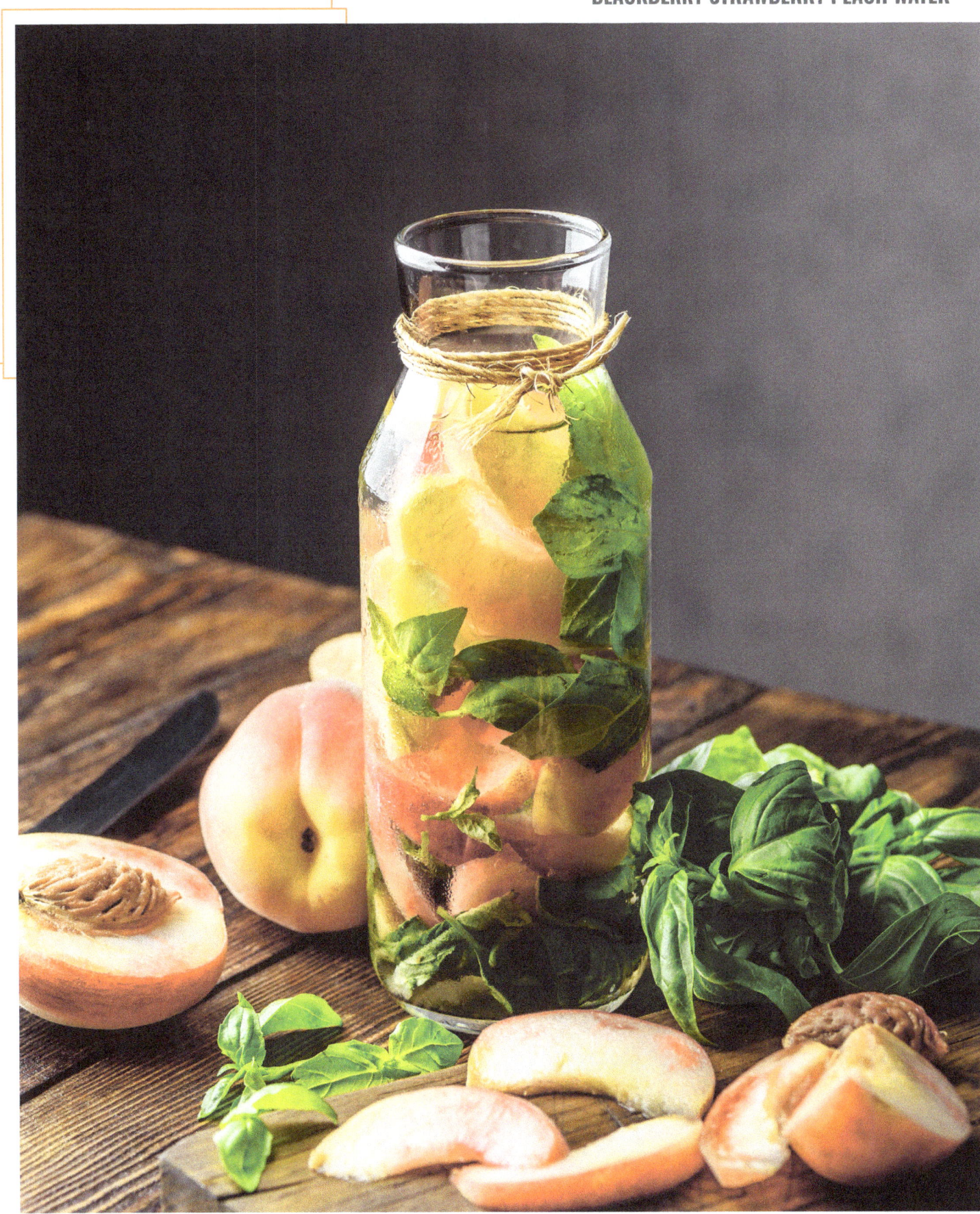

45

BLACKBERRY STRAWBERRY PEACH WATER

Benefits
- Improves heart and brain health
- Reduces inflammation
- Fight infections
- Boost immune system
- Helps improve skin

INGREDIENTS

- 3/4 cups Granulated date sugar
- 1½ cups Water
- 1 cup Blackberries
- 2 diced Peaches
- 1 1/2 ounces of water
- Ice cubes

INSTRUCTIONS

FOR SIMPLE SYRUP:
1. Pour 1 cup of water, date sugar, blackberries and peaches in a saucepan.
2. Cook them on a medium heat until they start to boil.
3. Reduce the heat to a simmer and then cook for more 10-15 minutes.
4. Set it aside to cool for 15-20 minutes.
5. Pass it through a fine mesh sieve and press the fruit against the side using a spatula.

TO MAKE ONE COCKTAIL:
6. Add some ice cubes in a cocktail shaker.
7. Pour in ¼ cup blackberry/peach simple syrup.
8. Then add 1/2 cup of water.
9. Blend them well to prepare the base of the drink.
10. Pour it into the glass and add some more ice if needed.

ORANGE KIWI WATER

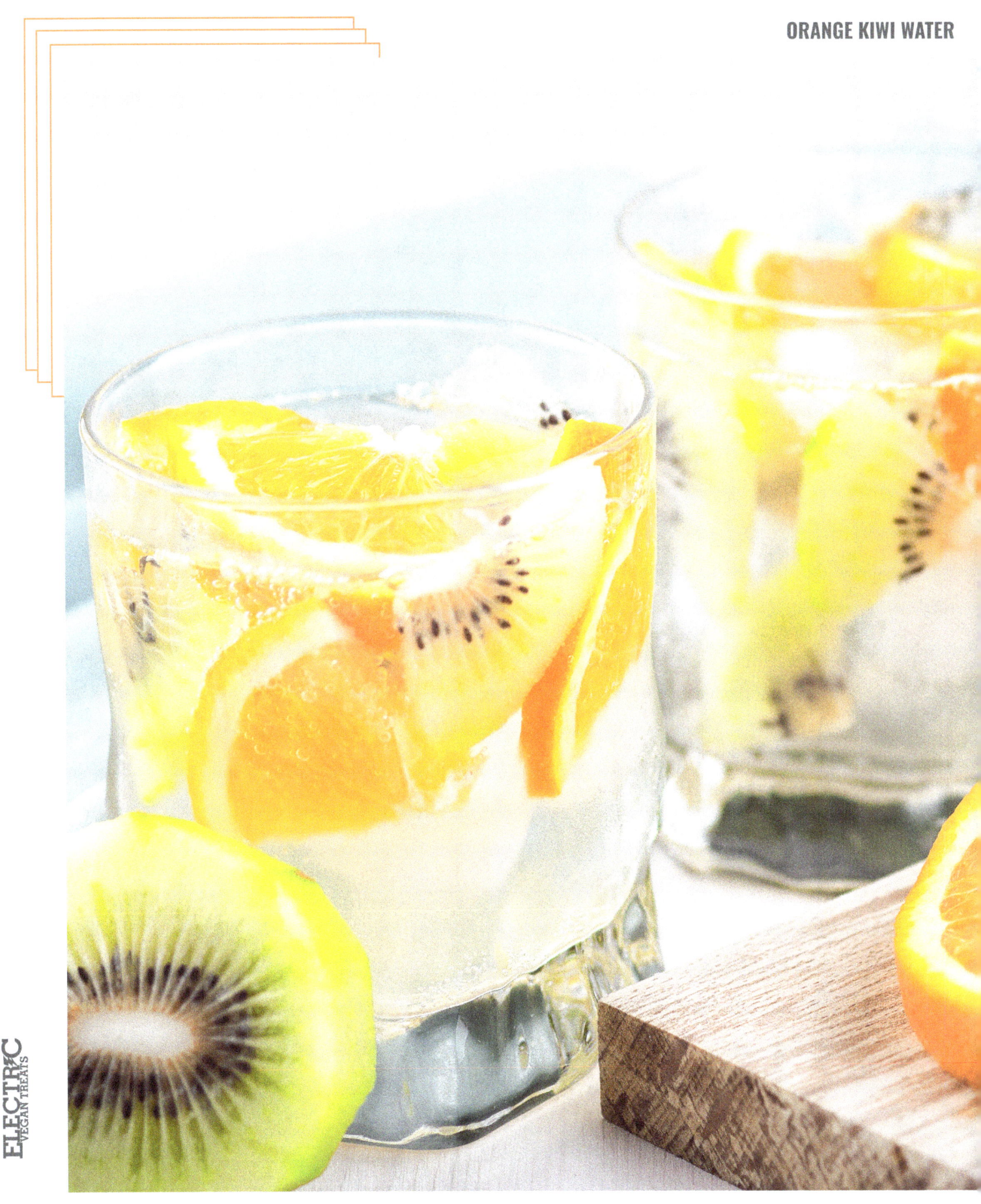

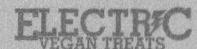

ORANGE KIWI WATER

Benefits

- Great source of fiber
- Helps lower cholesterol
- Aids Ulcer protection
- Helps prevent kidney
- Helps improve skin booster
- Helps improve eye health
- Aids in weight loss
- Rheumatoid arthritis relief

INGREDIENTS

- 1 ripe kiwi fruit
- 1/2 cup orange juice
- 2 teaspoon icing date sugar
- 12 ounces of water
- Ice cubes
- 1 slice orange cut into half for garnishing
- 1 slice kiwi cut into half for garnishing

INSTRUCTIONS

1. Grab a ripe kiwi, peel it and then cut it into chunks.
2. Mash it well as finely as you can.
3. Take 2 glasses or serving juice jars and place the kiwi at the bottom.
4. Pour 1/4 cup of orange juice on top of the kiwi in each glass.
5. Add 1 teaspoon of icing date sugar in each glass.
6. Pour some water to fill the glass and then mix it with a spoon.
7. Add some ice cubes in the each glass and serve it chilled.
8. Garnish with some orange and kiwi slices.

BLUEBERRY LIME WATER

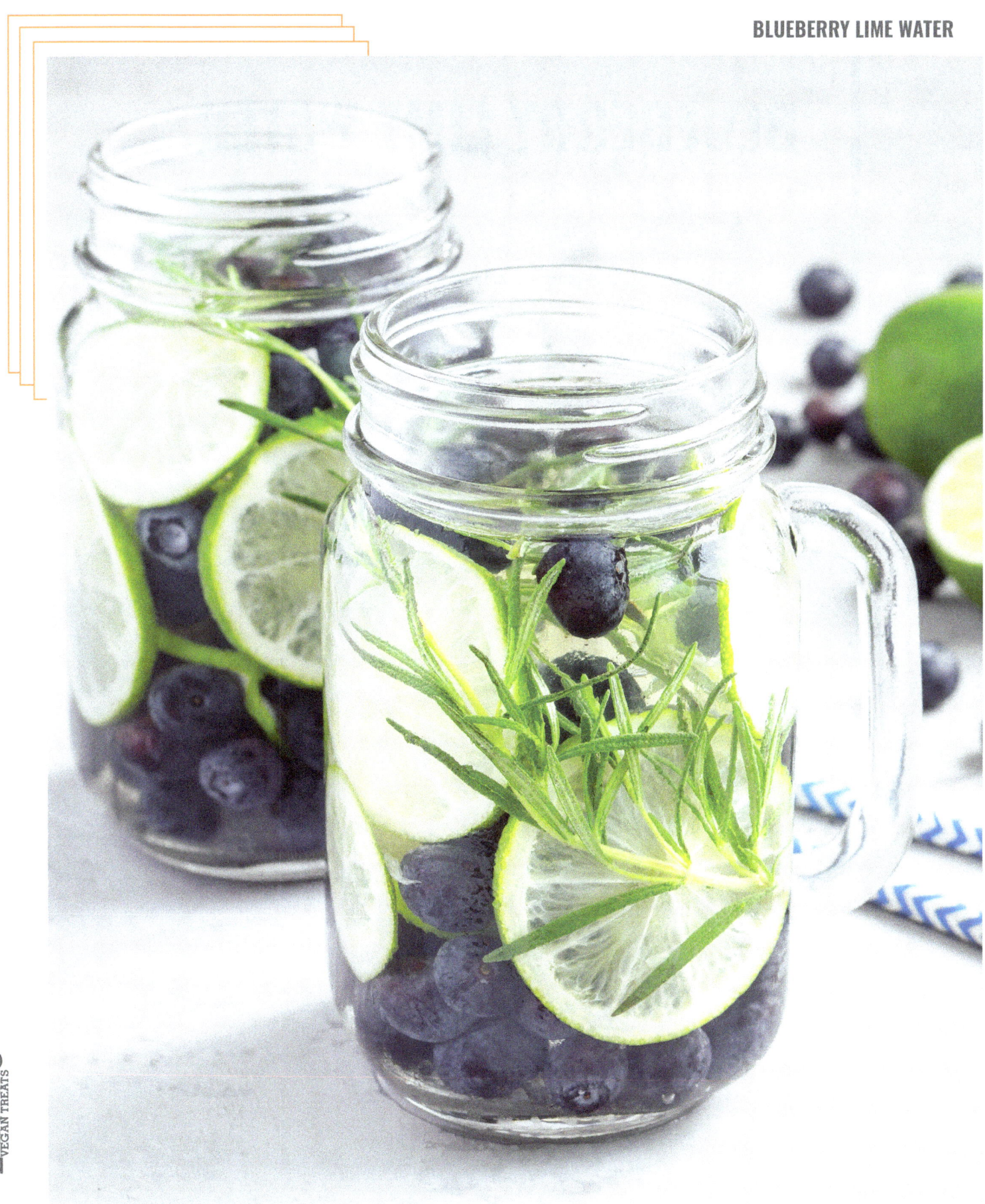

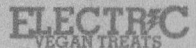

BLUEBERRY LIME WATER

Benefits

- Aids in bone health
- High in iron, phosphorous, calcium, magnesium, zinc, and vitamin K
- Improves skin
- Blood pressure control
- Helps improve diabetes
- Helps prevent heart disease
- Improves mental health

INGREDIENTS

- 2 cups fresh blueberries
- ½ cup granulated date sugar
- ⅓ cup lime juice
- 3 cups water or more if needed
- Ice cubes

INSTRUCTIONS

1. Grab a blender and combine blueberries, date sugar, lime juice, and 3 cups water.
2. More water can be added to achieve the desired consistency.
3. Add some ice cubes in the blender and pulse them well.
4. Transfer it to the glass and enjoy!

STRAWBERRY BASIL WATER

STRAWBERRY BASIL WATER

Benefits

- Detoxifying
- Hydrating
- Assists with weight loss
- Helps clear skin
- Full of vitamin C
- Anti-inflammatory
- Anti-oxidants
- Antibacterial
- Antimicrobial
- Anti-cancer

 ### INGREDIENTS

- 4 cups fresh strawberries
- 2 Freshly squeezed lemons
- 1 cup fresh basil
- Sparkling water

 ### INSTRUCTIONS

1. In a jug, combine strawberries, lemon juice, basil and water.
2. Let it infuse for some hours.
3. Add some sparkling water.
4. Put some ice cubes in the serving glass and then pour it over the ice.

WATERMELON CUCUMBER MINT WATER

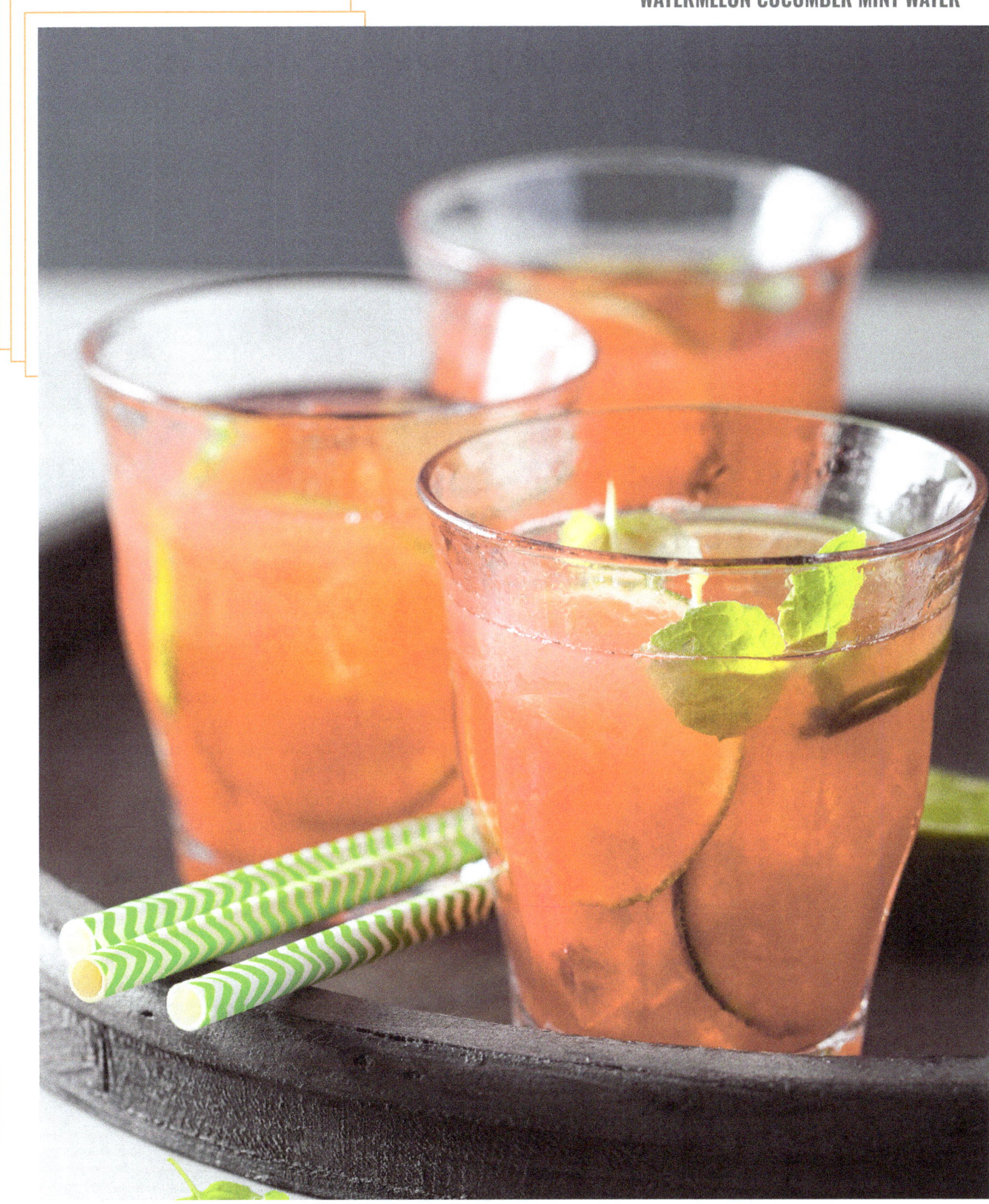

WATERMELON CUCUMBER MINT WATER

Benefits
- Anti-oxidants
- Antibacterial
- Antimicrobial
- Anti-cancer

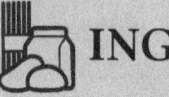 ## INGREDIENTS

- 1 medium sized peeled watermelon (cubed)
- 1 large peeled cucumber (diced)
- 1 1/2 cups fresh mint leaves
- 3 cups fresh water
- 1/2 cup cane date sugar
- Juice of a lemon

 ## INSTRUCTIONS

1. Grab a saucepan and combine the water and pure cane date sugar.
2. Boil them on medium-high heat and continue stirring until date sugar is fully dissolved.
3. Remove the saucepan from the stove, add the mint leaves to hot mixture.
4. Cover the saucepan and let it set for about half an hour.
5. Take a blender or food processor and pulse sliced watermelons and cucumber.
6. Add in lemon juice and blend them well for about 2 minutes until smooth.
7. Now add the pre-prepared mint infused water and again give it a good mix.
8. Strain the juice into the jar and chill in the refrigerator for about 2 hours.
9. Add some ice cubes in the glasses and pour the juice over it.
10. Garnish with some fresh mint leaf.

BLUEBERRY APPLE RASPBERRY WATER

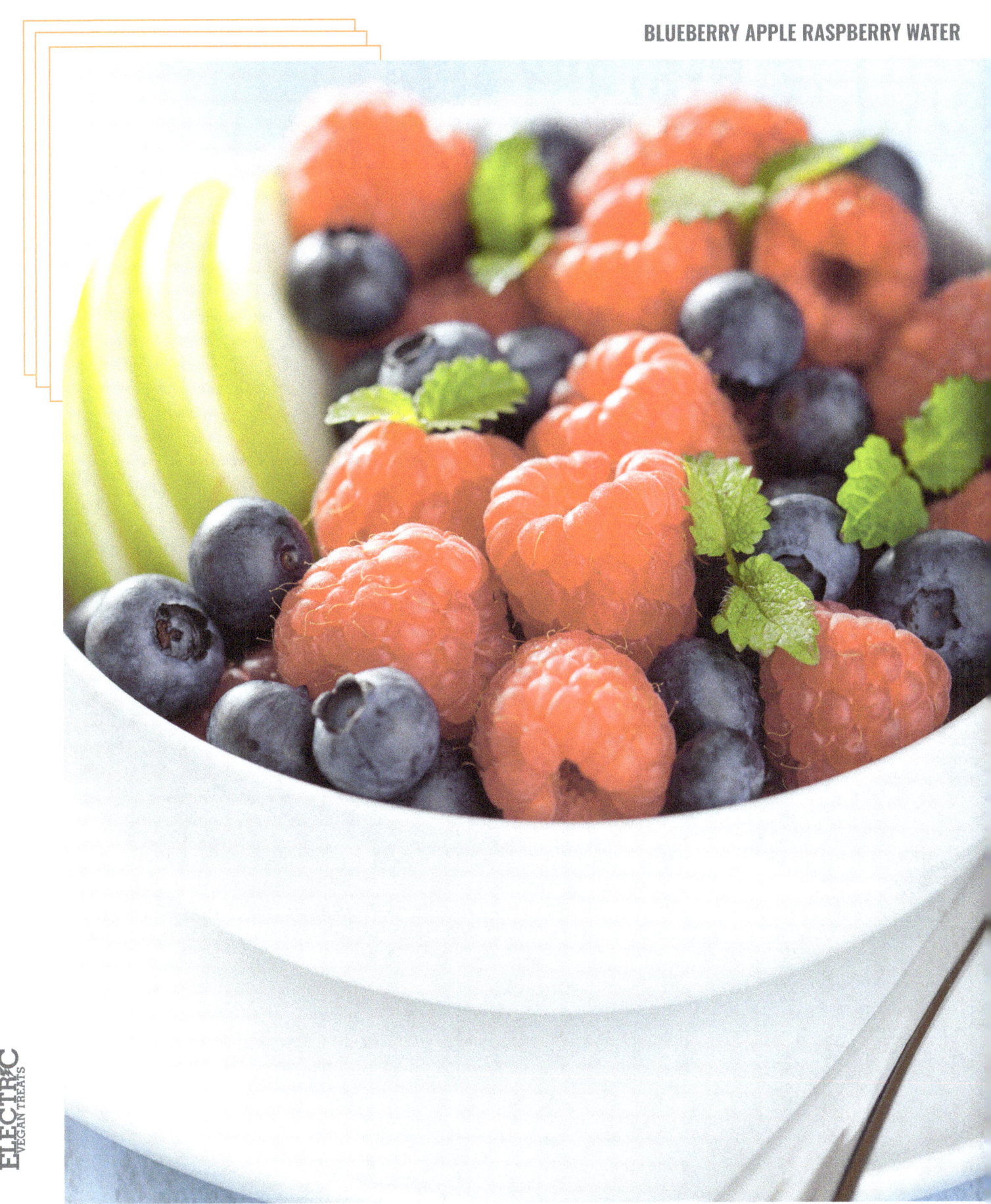

BLUEBERRY APPLE RASPBERRY WATER

Benefits

- High in antioxidants
- High in phytonutrients and vitamins
- Helps improve skin

INGREDIENTS

- 4 apples (cored and diced)
- 2 cups raspberry
- 1 cup blueberries
- 1 cucumber diced
- 2 cups spinach
- Water as required

INSTRUCTIONS

1. Take a blender, add all ingredients in it and blend them well.
2. Refrigerate it for at least 2 hours.
3. Pour it in serving glasses and enjoy!

LEMON THYME WATER

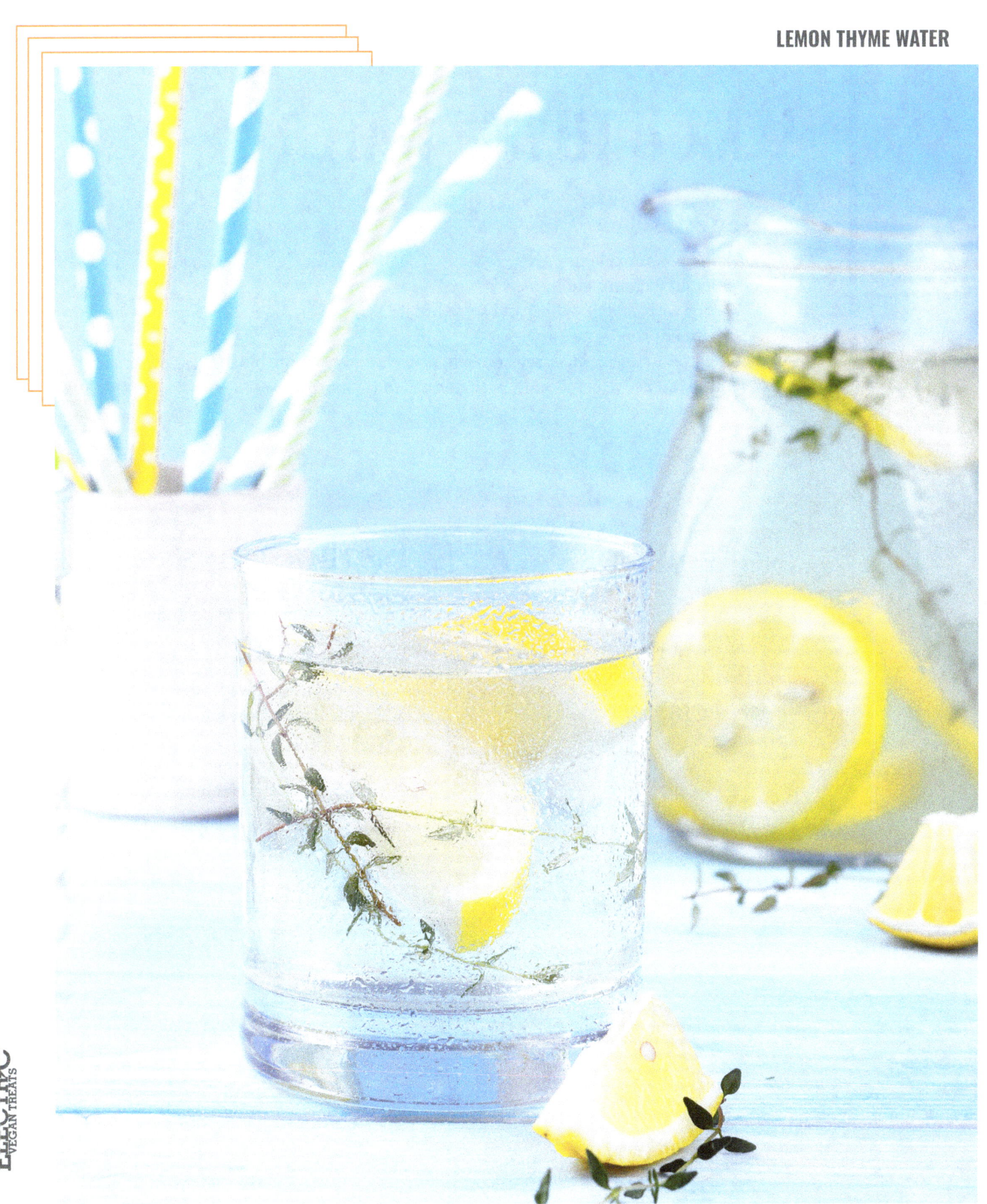

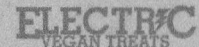

LEMON THYME WATER

Benefits

- High in antioxidants
- High in vitamins and minerals
- Helps with colds, coughs, and sore throat
- Helps improve acne
- Relieves indigestion, upset stomach, nausea, constipation, bloating, and cramping due to an active compound in thyme called thymol

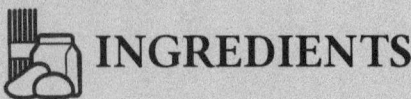

INGREDIENTS

- 1 1/2 cups date sugar
- 1 bunch fresh thyme
- 2 cups fresh lemon juice
- 5 cups water

INSTRUCTIONS

1. Grab a medium saucepan and add date sugar, thyme and 1 cup water.
2. Bring it to boil and keep stirring until the date sugar is dissolved.
3. Pour the lemon juice and add the remaining 4 cups of water.
4. Strain the juice in a jug.
5. Refrigerate for about 2 hours and serve over ice.

SUGGESTIONS:

1. Do not drink will pregnant. Do not drink if on thyroid medications, it may cause an adverse reaction.

CUCUMBER LIME STRAWBERRY MINT WATER

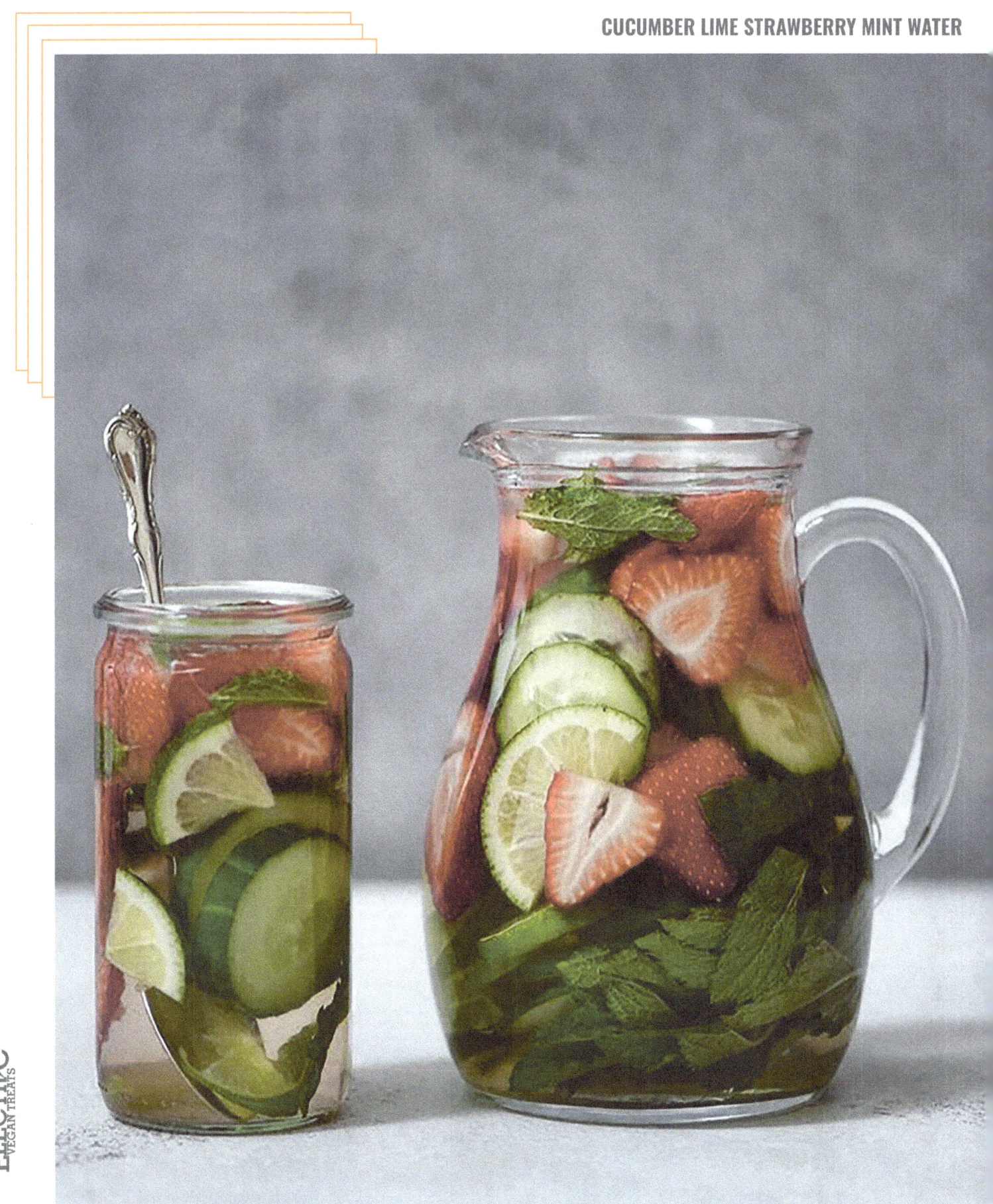

CUCUMBER LIME STRAWBERRY MINT WATER

Benefits
- Detoxifying
- Hydrating
- Improves skin
- Full of vitamins
- Anti-inflammatory properties
- Helps with weight loss

INGREDIENTS

- 1/2 sliced cucumber
- 1 cup sliced strawberries
- 1 sliced lime
- A handful of mint leaves
- 2 cups cold water

INSTRUCTIONS

1. Grab a large bowl and add all ingredients in it.
2. Fill it with cold water.
3. Cover the bowl and place it in fridge to infuse for at least one hour.

ORANGE STAR ANISE HIBISCUS WATER

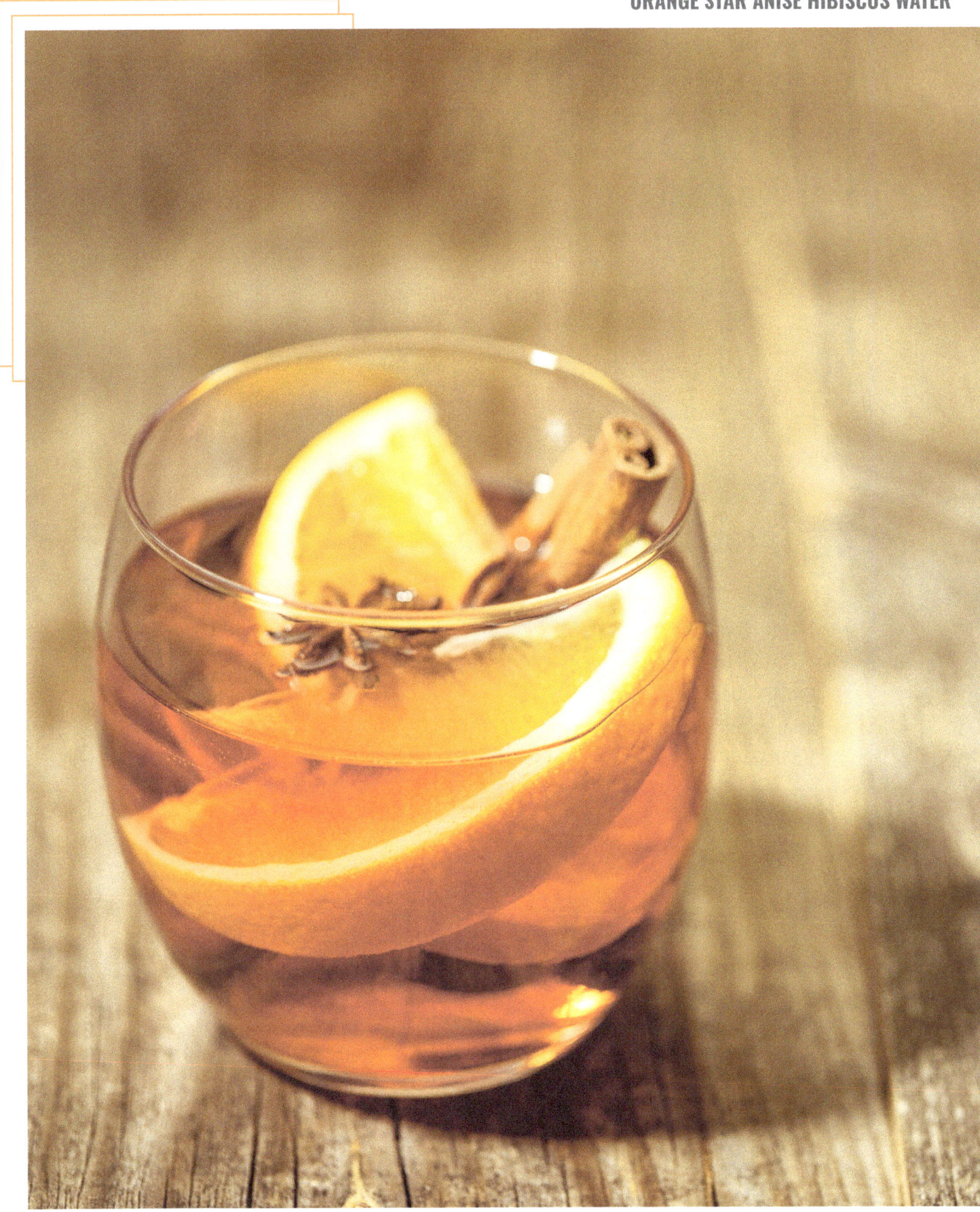

ORANGE STAR ANISE HIBISCUS WATER

Benefits

- Helps with weight lose
- Helps reduce cholesterol
- Good source of vitamin C

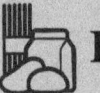 **INGREDIENTS**

- 2 large Dried hibiscus petals
- 2 cups Water
- 1 inch Ginger chopped
- 1 peeled and diced orange
- 5 star anise
- 2 teaspoon Agave

 **INSTRUCTIONS**

1. Grab a tea infuser and add hibiscus petals, star anise and ginger along with water.
2. Let them infuse for 3-4 hours.
3. Now add dices orange and honey in the end.
4. Mix them well with a wooden spoon.
5. Leave them for about 2 hours in the refrigerator.
6. Transfer to the cups and enjoy!

WATER MELON HONEYDEW AND MINT WATER

WATERMELON HONEYDEW MINT WATER

Benefits
- High in vitamin C
- Aids in weight-loss
- Great for pre and post workout
- A natural coolant

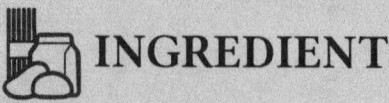 **INGREDIENTS**

- 1 cup date sugar
- 1 cup water
- Zest of 2 limes
- ⅓ cup mint leaves
- 2 cups chopped agavedew melon
- 1 cup fresh lime juice
- Diced watermelon (half)
- 3 cups cold water

 INSTRUCTIONS

1. Grab a saucepan and boil date sugar, 1 cup water, zest of 2 limes and mint leaves.
2. Keep stirring until everything combines well.
3. Let cool it cool for about an hour.
4. Now take a blender and add agavedew, fresh lime juice, diced watermelon and 3 cups cold water.
5. Add the mint date sugar mix and again blend it well.
6. Now transfer it to a jar and chill for about 2 hours.

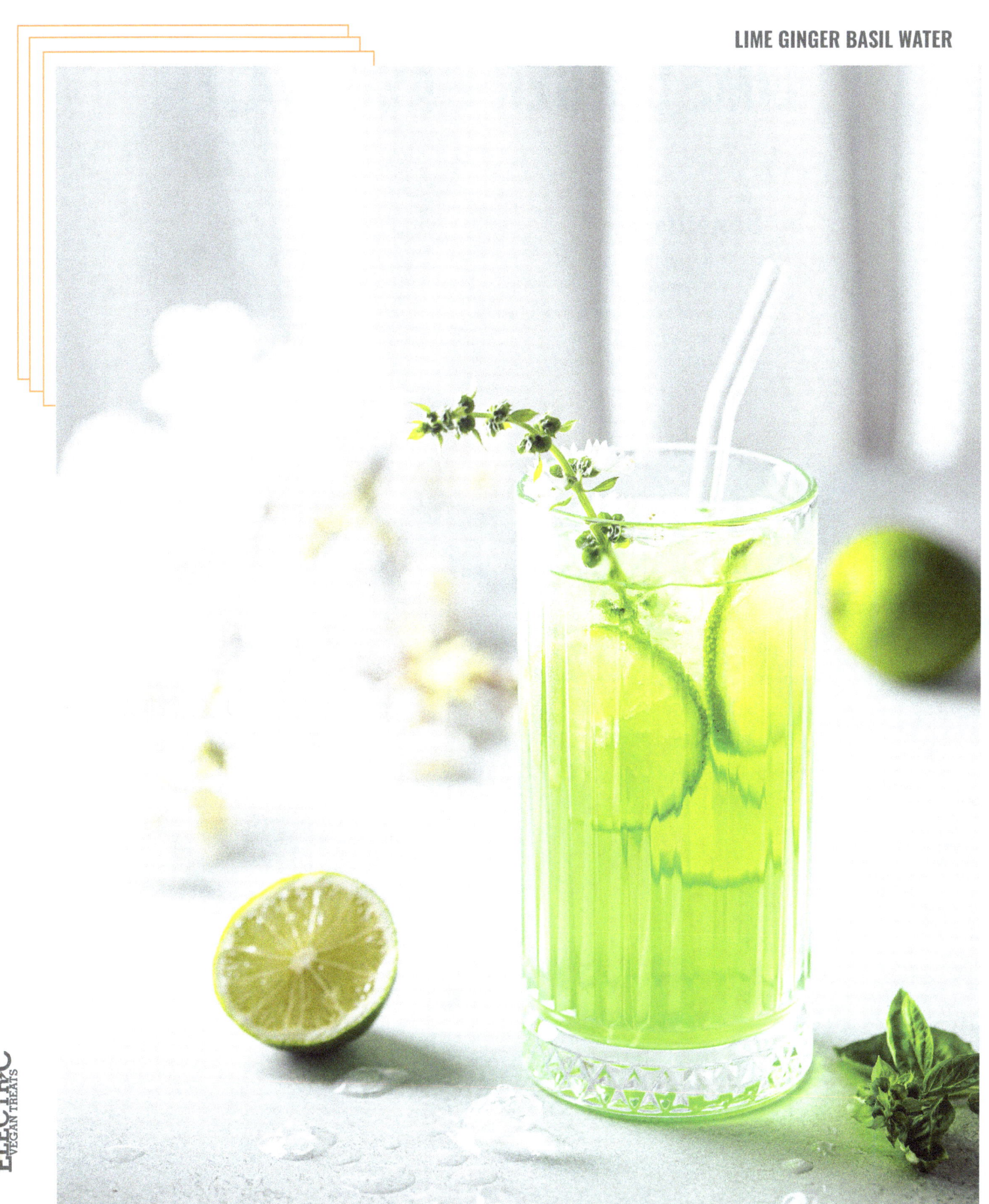

LIME GINGER BASIL WATER

LIME GINGER BASIL WATER

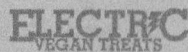

Benefits
- Anti-inflammatory
- Anti-nausea
- Improves gastrointestinal health
- Boost immune system
- Assist with cancer prevention

 ## INGREDIENTS

- 2 lemons
- 5 ginger pieces
- 3/4 cup basil leaves
- 3 tablespoons agave
- 9 cups boiling water

 ## INSTRUCTIONS

1. Cut the lemons into halves and squeeze them into a large pitcher.
2. Add the squeezed slices in the pitcher and avoid any seeds.
3. Now add the ginger pieces and basil leaves.
4. Pour the boiling water into the pitcher and then add the agave.
5. Stir in the agave and then leave it for about an hour to cool down.
6. Remove the ginger, basil, and lemon halves from the pitcher.
7. Refrigerate it until chilled well.
8. Transfer the infused water in serving glasses and serve with ice.

LEMON RASPBERRY ROSEMARY WATER

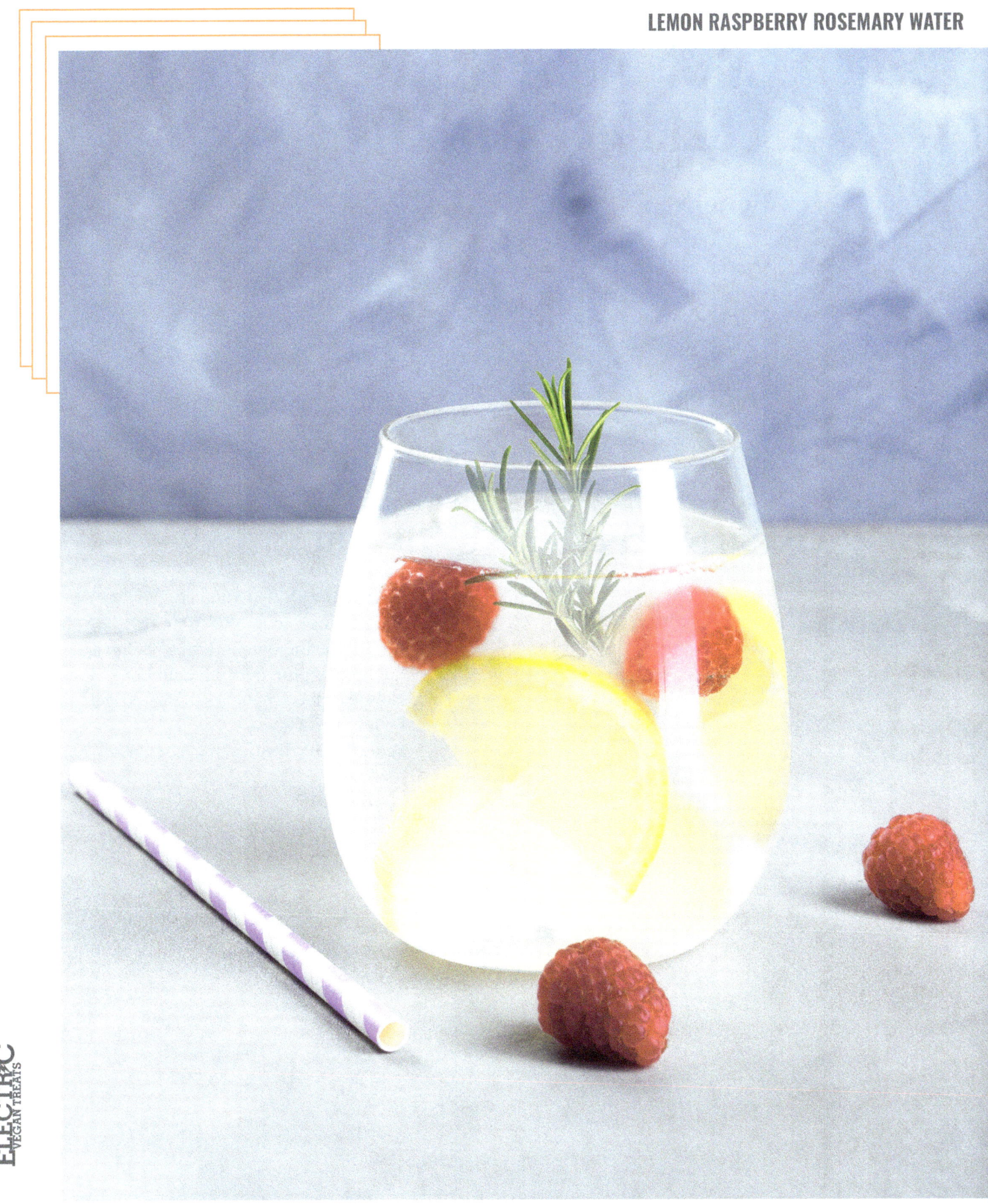

LEMON RASPBERRY ROSEMARY WATER

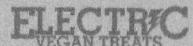

Benefits

- Hydrating
- Antioxidants
- High in vitamins
- Helps eliminate toxins
- Helps boost metabolism

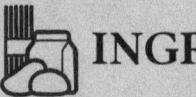 **INGREDIENTS**

- 16 fresh raspberries
- 6 lemon
- 2 small rosemary sprigs
- Water

 **INSTRUCTIONS**

1. Grab a cutting board and cut the raspberries and lemons into fine small slices.
2. Add all the ingredients into a pitcher and then cover it for at least 2 hours.
3. Now transfer the pitcher to the refrigerator for another 2 hours.
4. Serve it chilled with some ice cubes.

ORANGE BLUEBERRY BASIL WATER

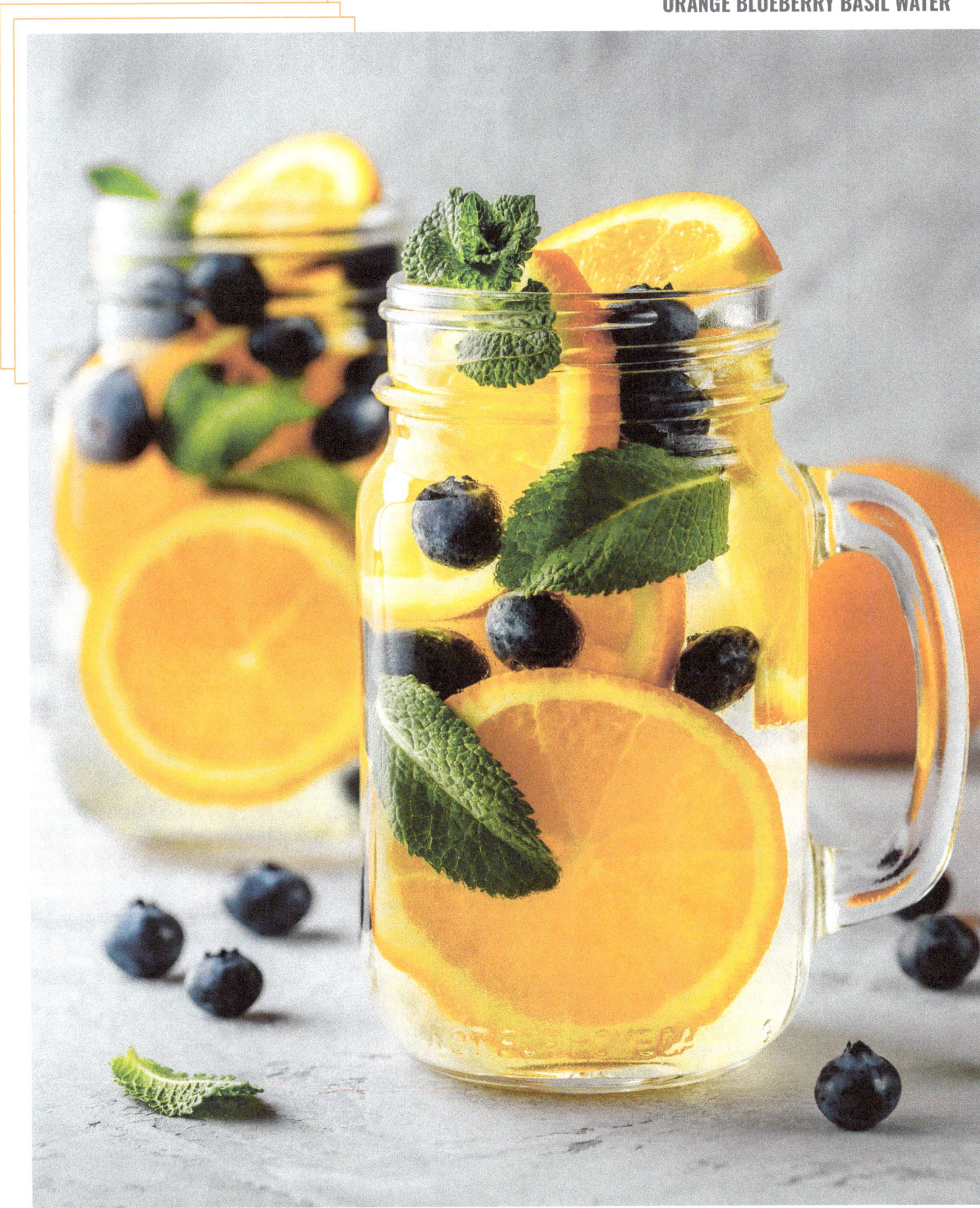

ORANGE BLUEBERRY BASIL WATER

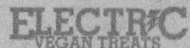

Benefits
- Hydrating
- High in vitamin C
- High in antioxidants

 ## INGREDIENTS

- 2 oranges
- ½ cup Blueberries
- 4 large fresh basil leaves
- 32 ounces chilled water

 ## INSTRUCTIONS

1. Peel off the oranges and cut them in slices.
2. Grab a bowl and add the orange slices along with the orange peel.
3. Now add the blueberries and basil leaves.
4. Mash the berries and orange slices gently by using a large spoon.
5. Add the chilled water to fill the bowl and cover it for a couple of hours.
6. Also, place it in the refrigerator to chill.
7. Serve with some ice cubes.

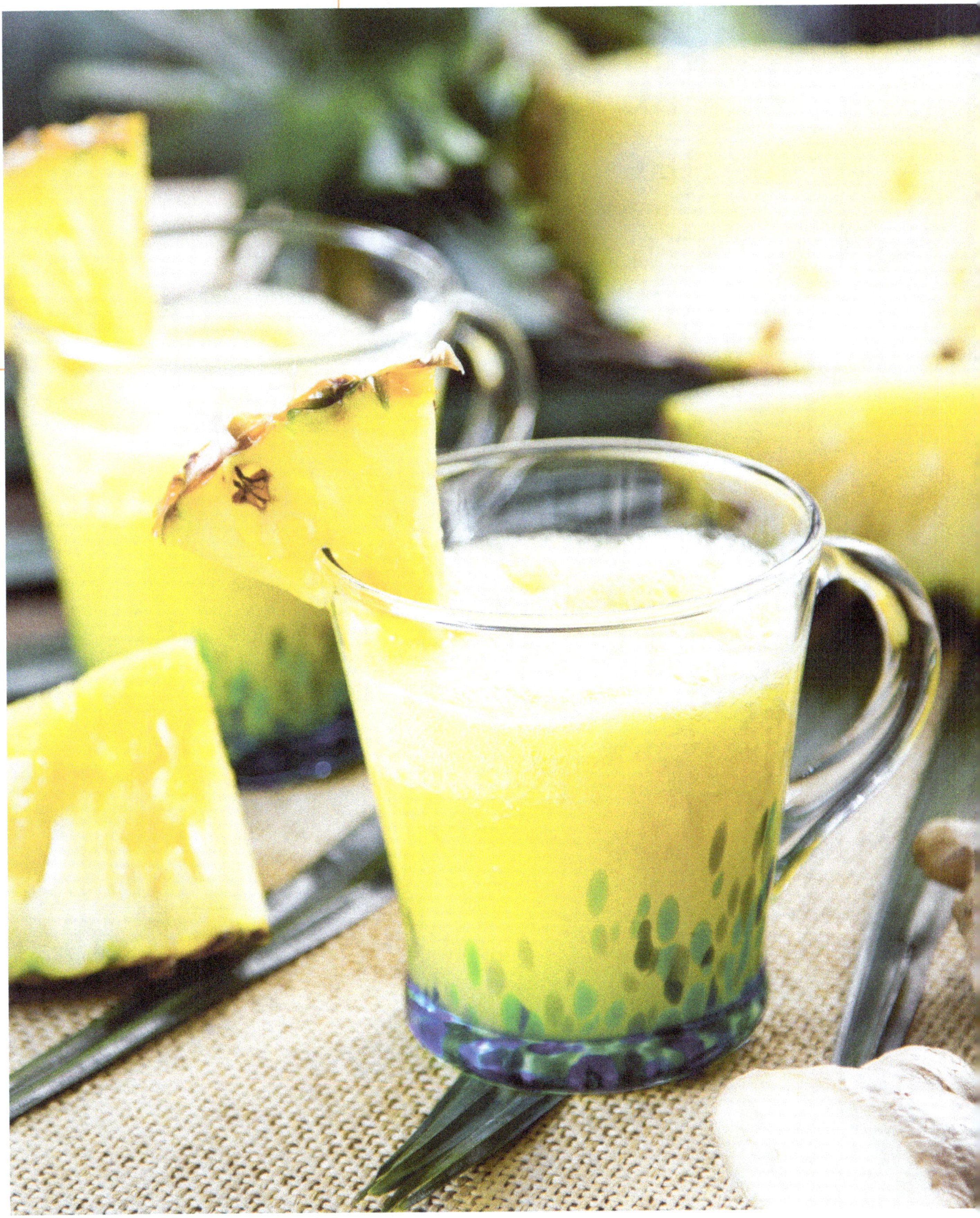

GINGER PINEAPPLE APPLE WATER

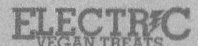

GINGER PINEAPPLE APPLE WATER

Benefits
- Aids in weight-loss
- Hydration,
- Assist with nausea and vomiting
- High in vitamin C

 INGREDIENTS

- ½ pineapple
- 1 apple
- 2-inches ginger
- 6 mint leaves
- 1 tablespoon agave
- 1/2 teaspoon salt
- Water

 INSTRUCTIONS

1. Peel and cut the pineapple, apple and ginger.
2. Add them in a blender along with mint leaves, salt and agave.
3. Give them a good mix.
4. Adjust the water quantity as per the requirement and consistency.
5. Strain it through a sieve and pour in the glasses.
6. Serve it chilled with ice cubes.

STRAWBERRY BLUEBERRY WATER

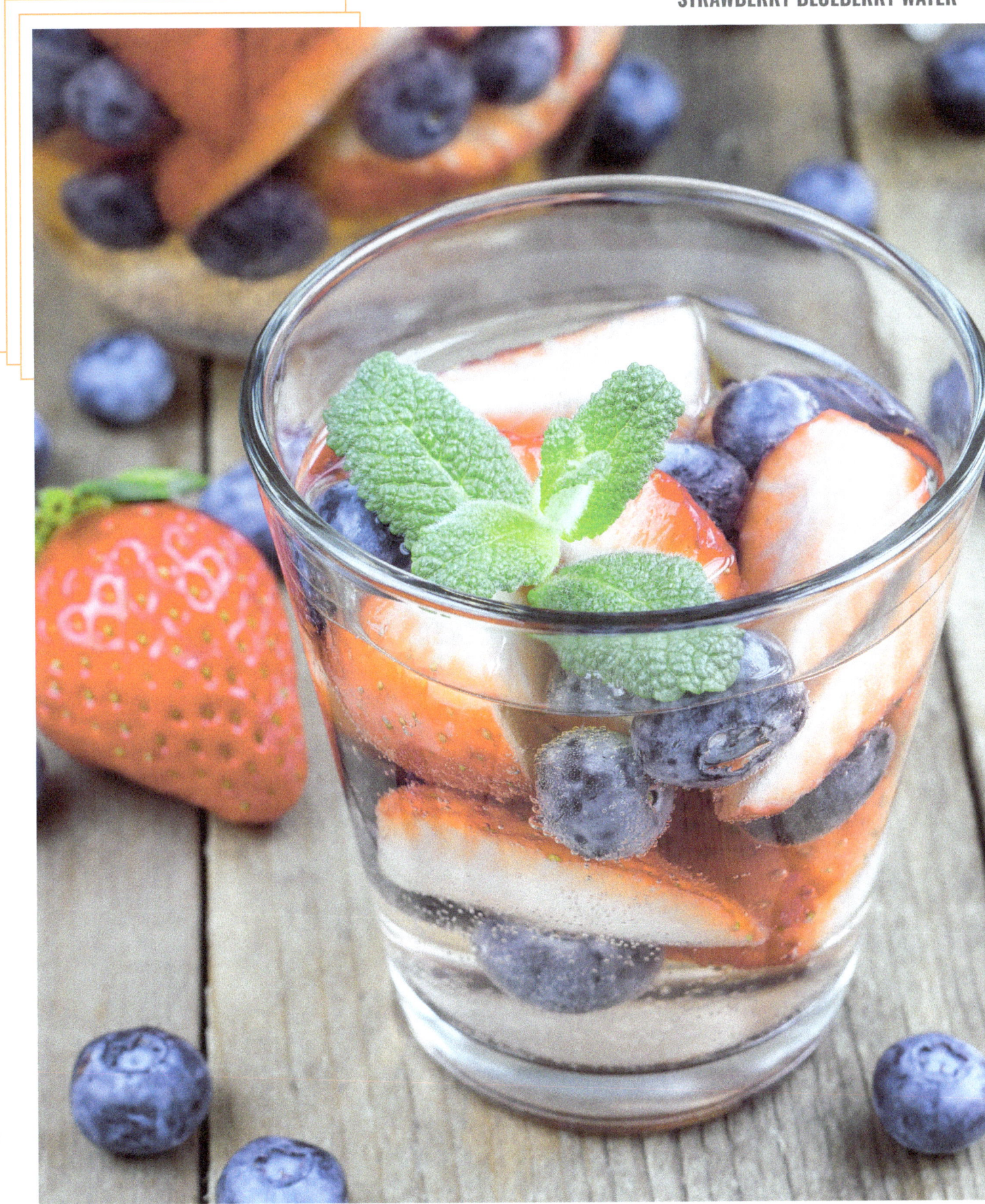

73

STRAWBERRY BLUEBERRY WATER

Benefits

- Aids in weight loss
- Full of antioxidants
- Loaded with vitamins
- Anti-aging properties
- Promotes brain health
- Anti-cancer properties

 ## INGREDIENTS

- 1 Cup Strawberries
- 1 Cup Blueberries
- 8 cups Water
- 1 cup Ice

 ## INSTRUCTIONS

1. Wash the strawberries and blueberries and pat them to dry.
2. Cut them into small slices and transfer them to a large pitcher.
3. Gently mash them with a large spoon so that they release some juice.
4. Now fill the pitcher with water, cover it and put into the refrigerator to infuse.
5. Wait for a few hours and transfer it to serving glasses.
6. Add ice to glasses and enjoy!

STRAWBERRY PINEAPPLE WATER

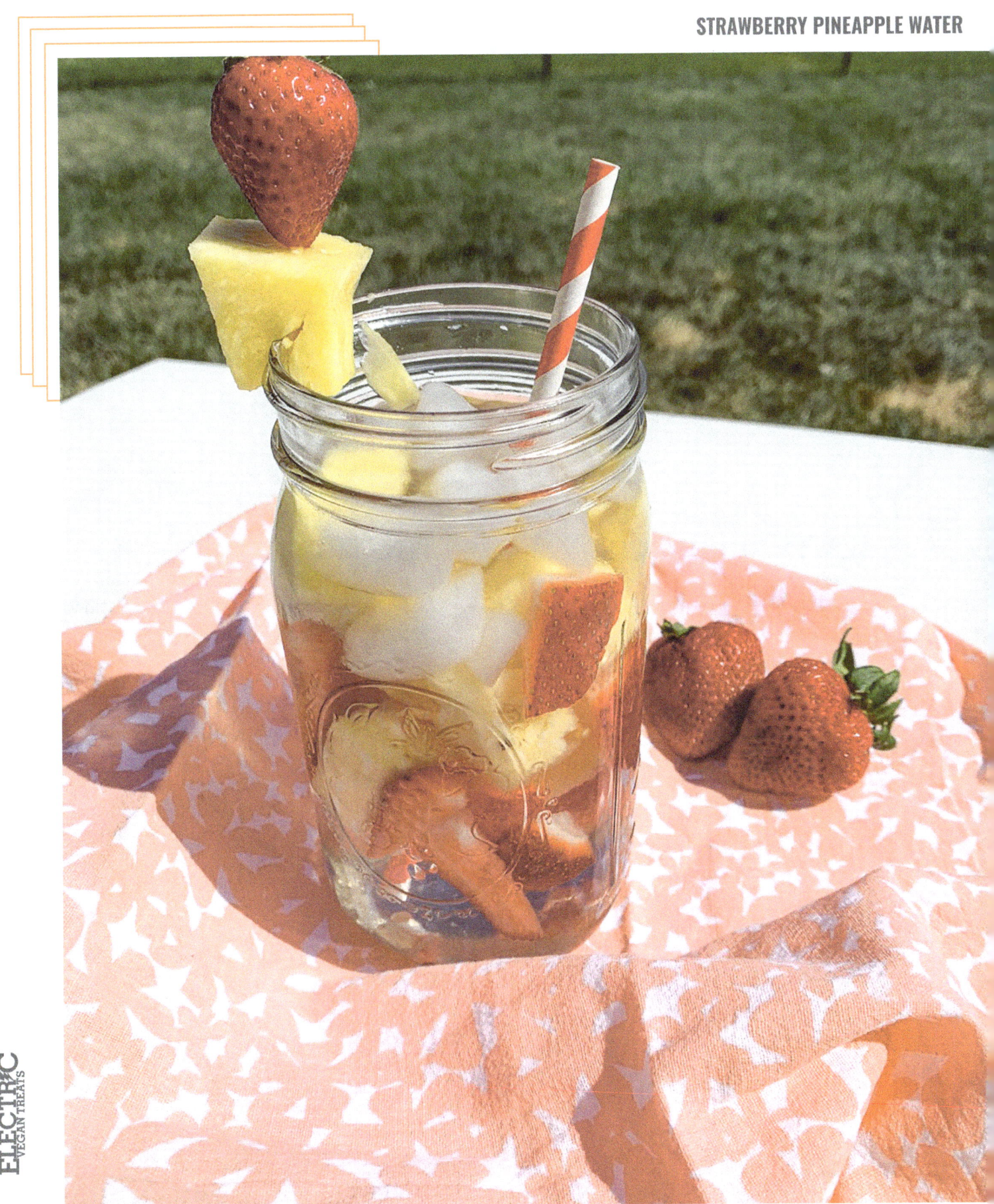

STRAWBERRY PINEAPPLE WATER

Benefits

- Detoxifying
- Hydrating
- Helps maintain teeth and bones
- High in electrolytes

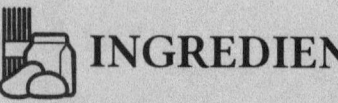 INGREDIENTS

- 2 cups fresh strawberries
- 4 cups fresh pineapple chunks
- 1/4 cup lemon juice
- 1 1//2 cup water
- 1 cup strawberries chunks for garnishing
- Ice
- lime wedges for garnishing

 INSTRUCTIONS

1. Grab a blender and combine the strawberries, pineapple chunks, lime juice, and 1 cup of water.
2. Blend them well until all the fruit has been combined perfectly.
3. Transfer the prepared puree to a jar and pass it through a sieve.
4. Now chill it in the refrigerator for at least 2 hours.
5. Pour in the serving glasses along with some ice and garnish some strawberry chunks and lime wedges.

ORANGE BLUEBERRY WATER

ORANGE BLUEBERRY WATER

Benefits

- High in Vitamin C
- Aids in weight loss
- High in antioxidants
- Loaded with vitamins
- Anti-aging properties
- Promotes brain health
- Anti-cancer properties
- Helps prevent UTIs
- Promotes heart health
- Anti-diabetic properties
- Helps with digestion
- Lowers blood pressure

 ## INGREDIENTS

- 6 cups water
- 2 oranges cut into wedges
- 1 bowl of fresh blueberries
- Ice cubes

 ## INSTRUCTIONS

1. Grab a pitcher and combine orange wedges and blueberries.
2. Mash them well with a large spoon and squeeze the orange wedges a bit.
3. Pour the water in the pitcher and put it the refrigerator for 4 hours.
4. Add some ice cubes at the bottom of the serving glasses and pour the prepared infused water.

APRICOT BERRIES MINT WATER

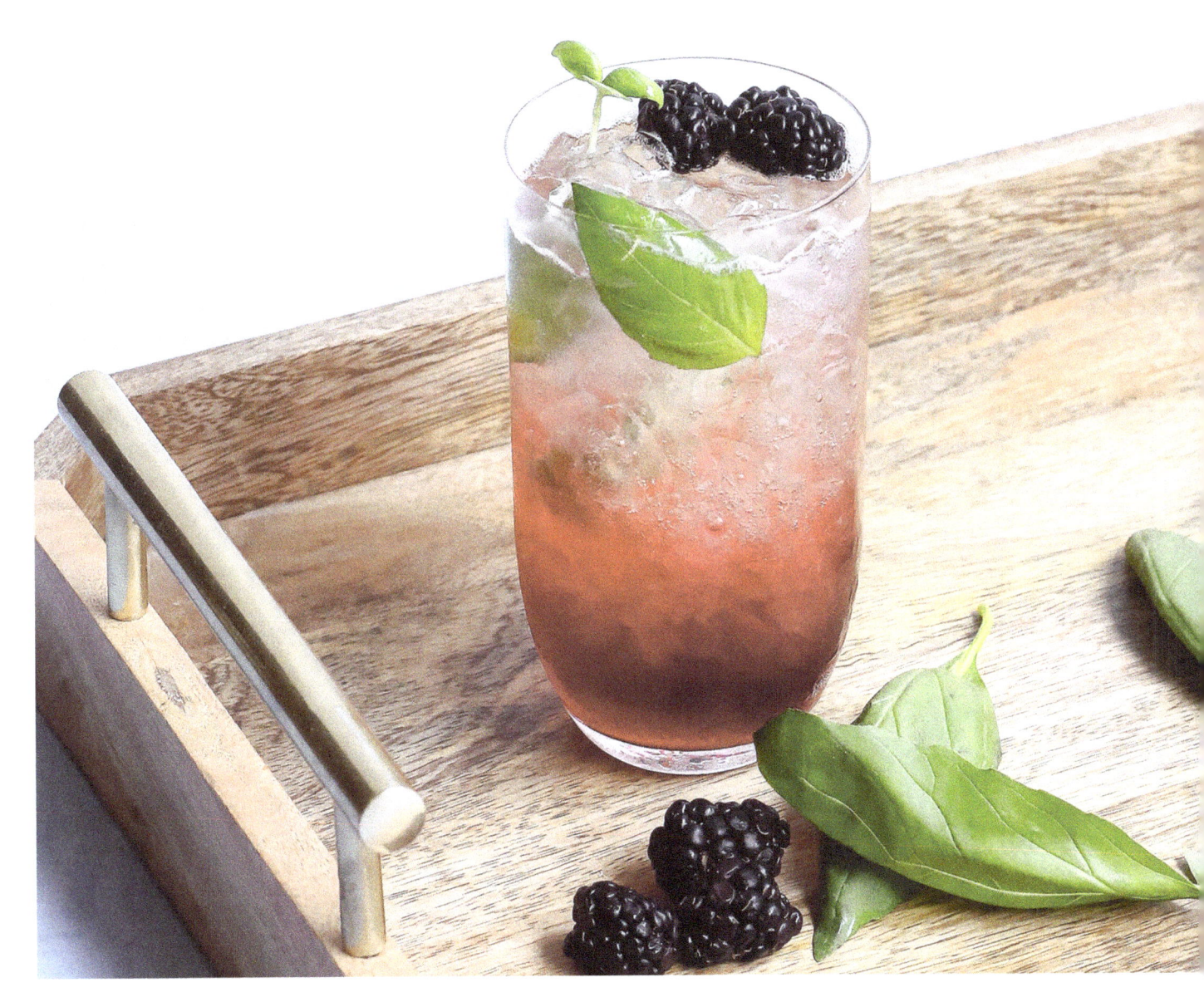

APRICOT MINT BERRIES WATER

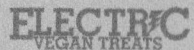

Benefits
- High in vitamin A
- Helps improve digestion
- Helps maintain strong bones
- Improves cardiovascular health
- High in potassium, vitamin C, and dietary fiber
- Helps reduces chances of heart attacks, strokes, and atherosclerosis

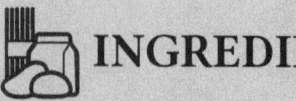 

INGREDIENTS

- 6 cups water
- 2 cups of fresh blueberries
- 8 mint sprigs
- 3 cups of apricot nectar
- Mint sprigs and apricot wedges for garnishing

INSTRUCTIONS

1. Grab a large saucepan and boil 3 cups of the water.
2. Remove from heat and add the mint springs in it.
3. Let it cool for a while.
4. Take a blender and combine the blueberries and apricot nectar to make a smooth puree.
5. Now transfer this puree to a large pitcher along with 3 cups of water.
6. Add the pre-heated mint water in the pitcher and give them a good mix.
7. Pass it through a sieve and chill for at least 4 hours.
8. Serve with some ice cubes and enjoy!

PEACH PLUM MINT WATER

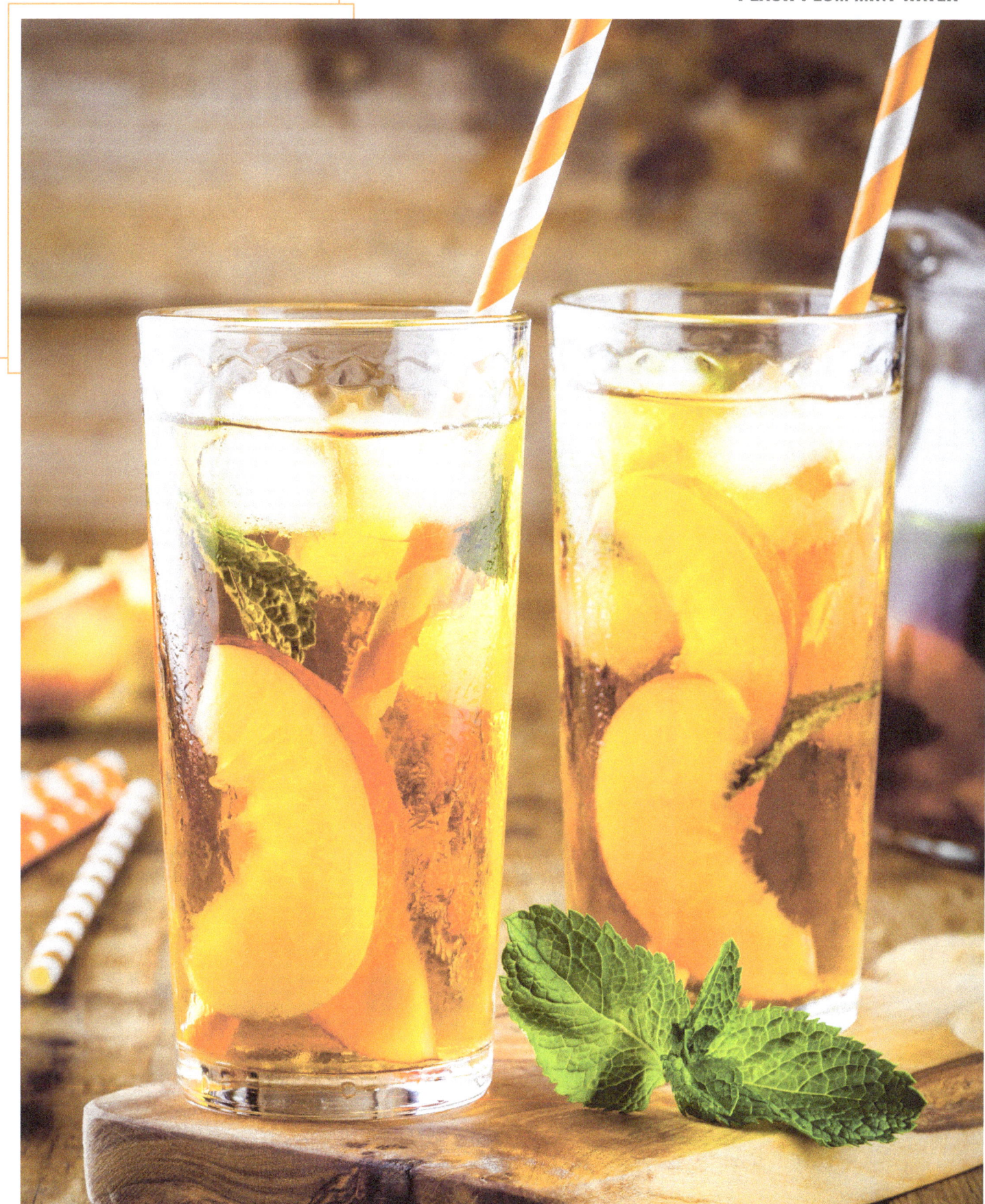

PEACH PLUM MINT WATER

Benefits
- High in fiber
- High in vitamin A,C,K, potassium, copper, and manganese
- Helps relives constipation
- High in antioxidants
- Helps lower blood sugar
- Helps promotes bone health

INGREDIENTS

- 6-8 plums
- 4 peaches
- 2 fresh mint leaves
- 1 pinch salt
- 1 cup Water
- Ice cubes

INSTRUCTIONS

1. Blend the plum and peaches in a blender.
2. Add a pinch of salt and a cup of water,
3. Give them a good mix.
4. Transfer it to a pitcher and add the mint leaves.
5. Cover the pitcher and leave it for at least 4 hours.
6. Pass it through a sieve and discard any solids and mint leaves.
7. Now refrigerate it for 2 hours and serve it chilled along with some ice cubes.

APPLE CINNAMON PEAR WATER

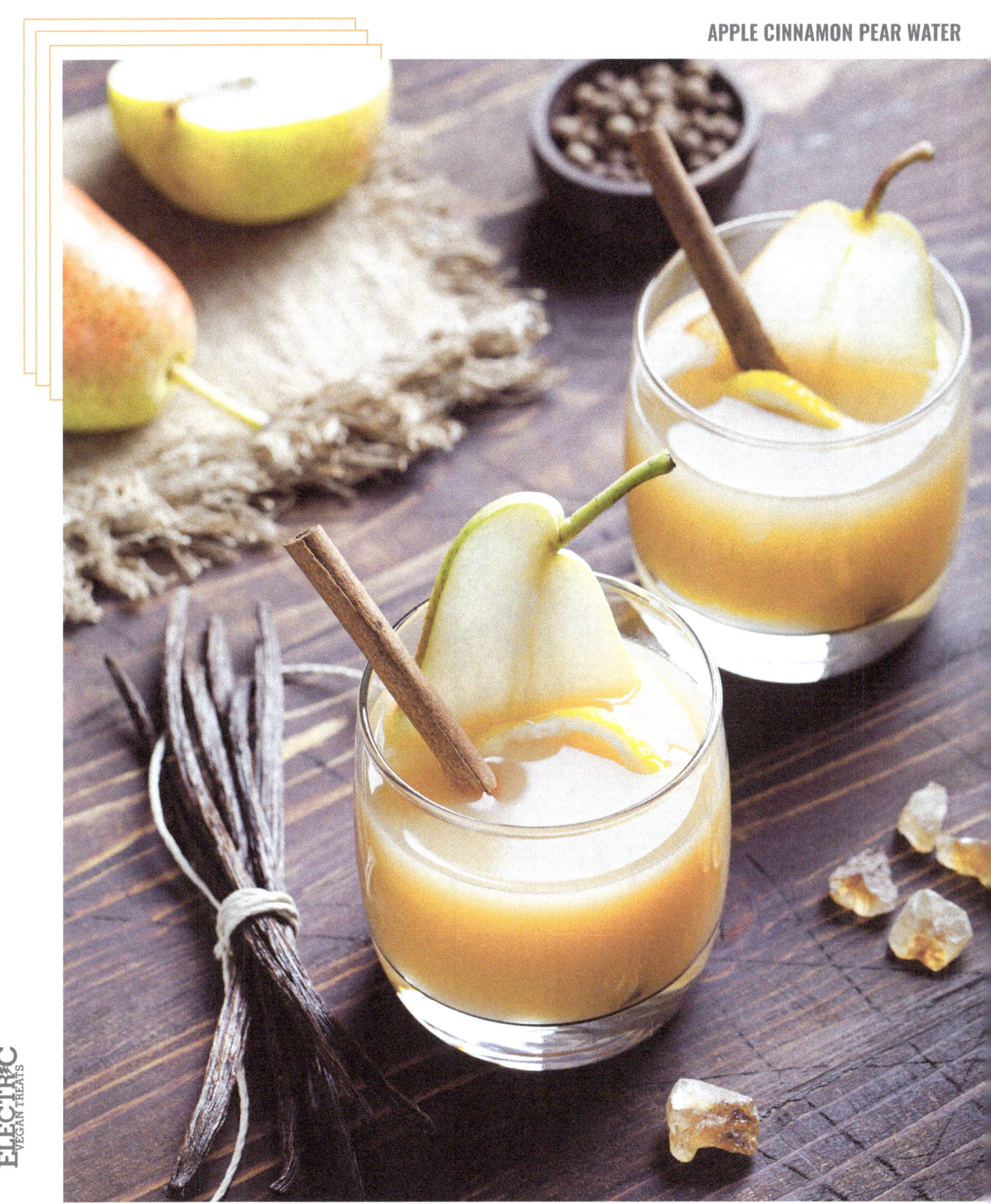

APPLE CINNAMON PEAR WATER

Benefits
- Anti-viral
- Anti-bacterial
- Anti-fungal properties
- Antioxidants
- Prebiotic properties
- Reduces blood pressure
- Lowers blood sugar
- Helps relieves digestive discomfort

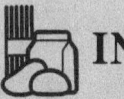 ## INGREDIENTS

- 1/2 apple
- 1 pear
- 2 small cinnamon sticks
- 4 cups of cold water

 ## INSTRUCTIONS

1. Boil 4 cups of water and pour it into a large pitcher.
2. Cut thin slices of apple and pear and place them in the pitcher.
3. Add the cinnamon sticks and cover the pitcher for an hour.
4. After an hour transfer the pitcher to the refrigerator and let it chill for at least 3 hours.

APPLE ORANGE CINNAMON CLOVE WATER

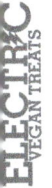

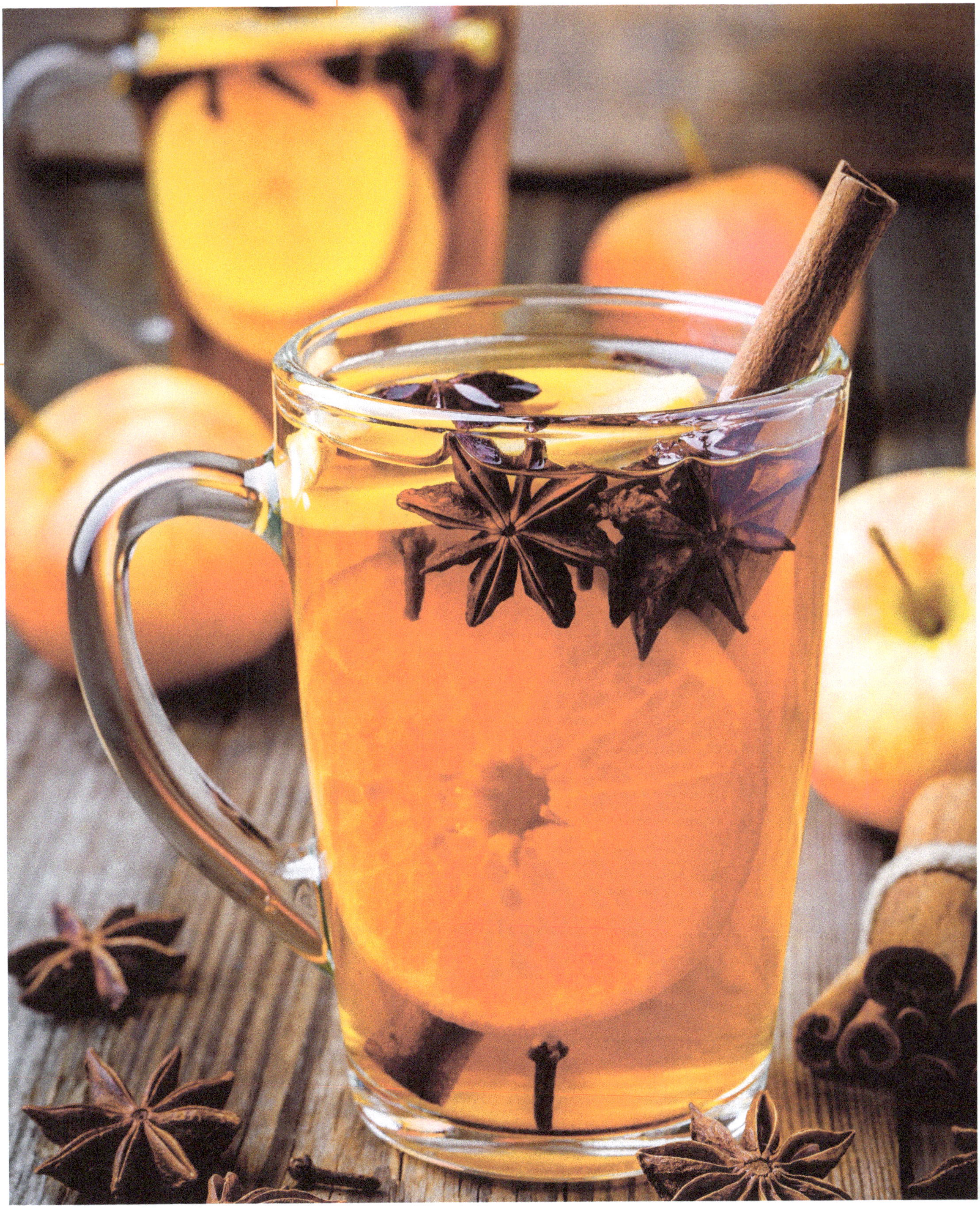

85

APPLE ORANGE CINNAMON CLOVE WATER

Benefits
- Great for fall
- High in antioxidants
- High in vitamins and minerals
- Helps curve appetite
- Helps regulate blood sugar
- Good for bone health
- High in vitamin C

INGREDIENTS

- 1/2 orange
- 1 small apple
- 4 cinnamon sticks
- 3 cloves
- 2 cups water

INSTRUCTIONS

1. Wash the orange and apple and pat them to dry.
2. Now cut them into small slices.
3. Blend the orange and apple with 2 cups of water.
4. Transfer them to a pitcher and add the cinnamon and cloves.
5. Cover the pitcher and place it in the refrigerator for 4 hours or overnight.

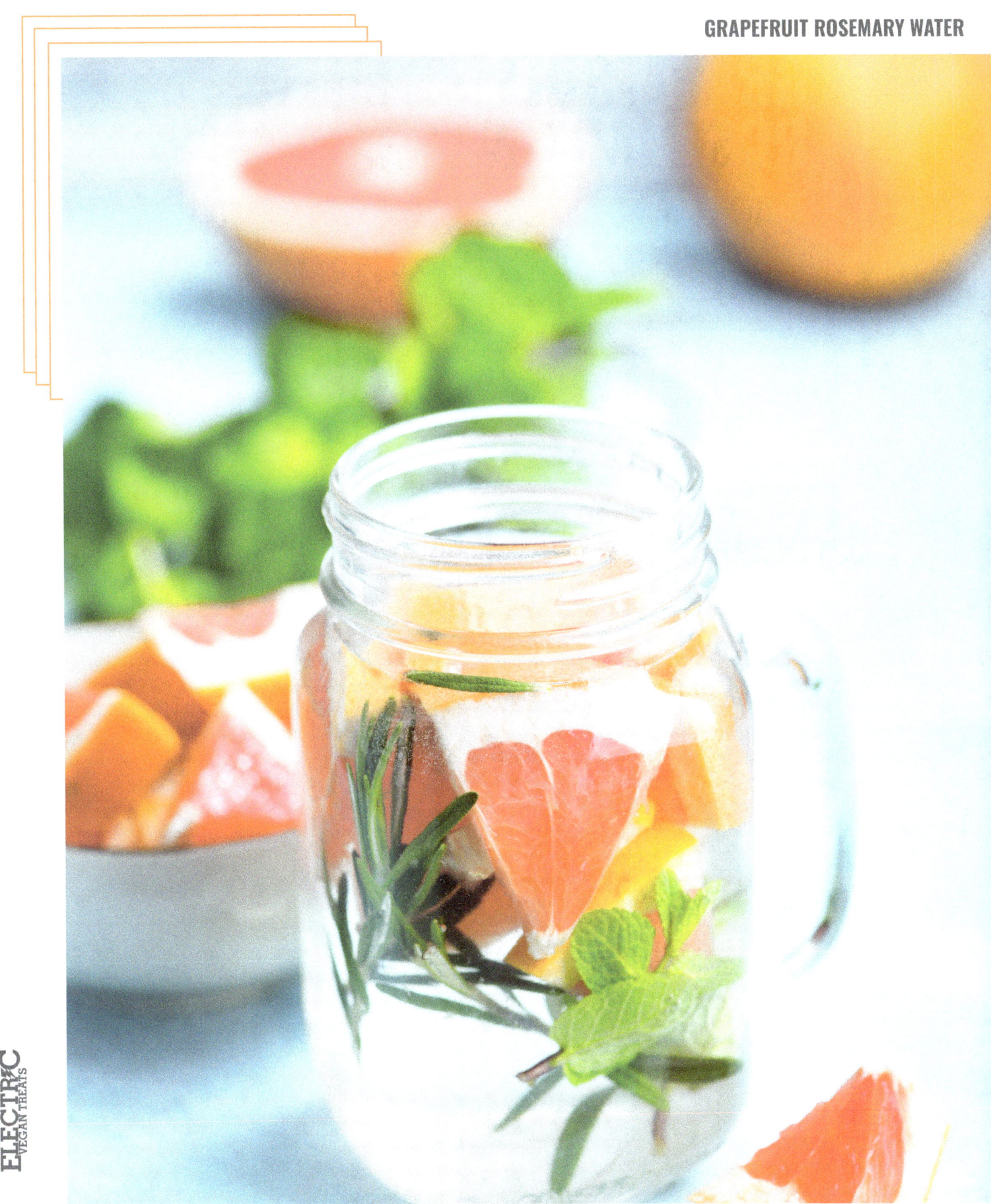
GRAPEFRUIT ROSEMARY WATER

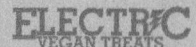

GRAPEFRUIT ROSEMARY WATER

Benefits

- Detoxifying
- Helps improve your mood, brain, and eye health
- Has small amounts of B vitamins, zinc, Cooper, and iron
- Helps you stay hydrated
- High in nutrients like fiber, protein, vitamin A and C, potassium, thiamine, folate, magnesium, antioxidants, and fiber
- Helps with weight-loss
- Helps boost your immune system

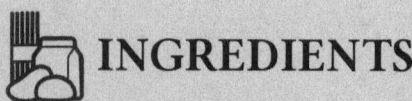

INGREDIENTS

- 1 grapefruits
- 10 sprigs of fresh rosemary
- 1 cups of water

INSTRUCTIONS

1. Cut the grapefruit into thin slices.
2. Place the grapefruit slices and rosemary at the bottom of a medium sized pitcher.
3. Fill the pitcher with a cup of water.
4. Refrigerate it for 2 hours and then transfer it to a glass filled with ice cubes.

CUCUMBER THYME LIME WATER

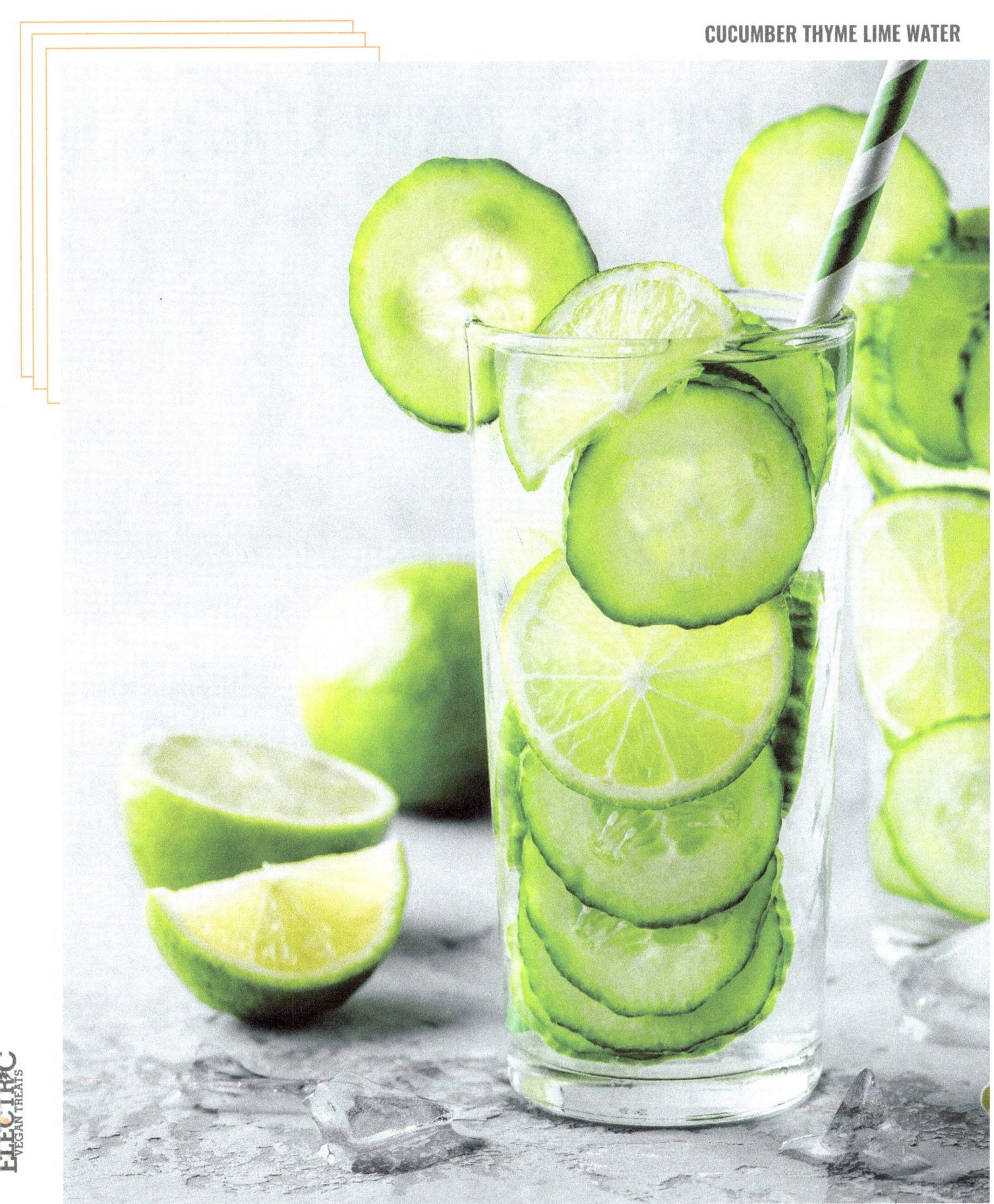

CUCUMBER THYME LIME WATER

Benefits
- High in nutrients
- Contains antioxidants
- Promotes hydration
- Promotes weight-loss
- helps lower blood sugar
- High in vitamin C

INGREDIENTS

- 1/2 cucumber
- 1 lime
- 2 rosemary sprigs
- A handful of thyme and mint

INSTRUCTIONS

1. Slice the cucumber and lime into small pieces.
2. Grab a pitcher and fill it with water.
3. Add the lime and cucumber slices along with rosemary springs and both herbs.
4. Refrigerate it for 2-4 hours before serving.

CRANBERRY AND ORANGE WATER

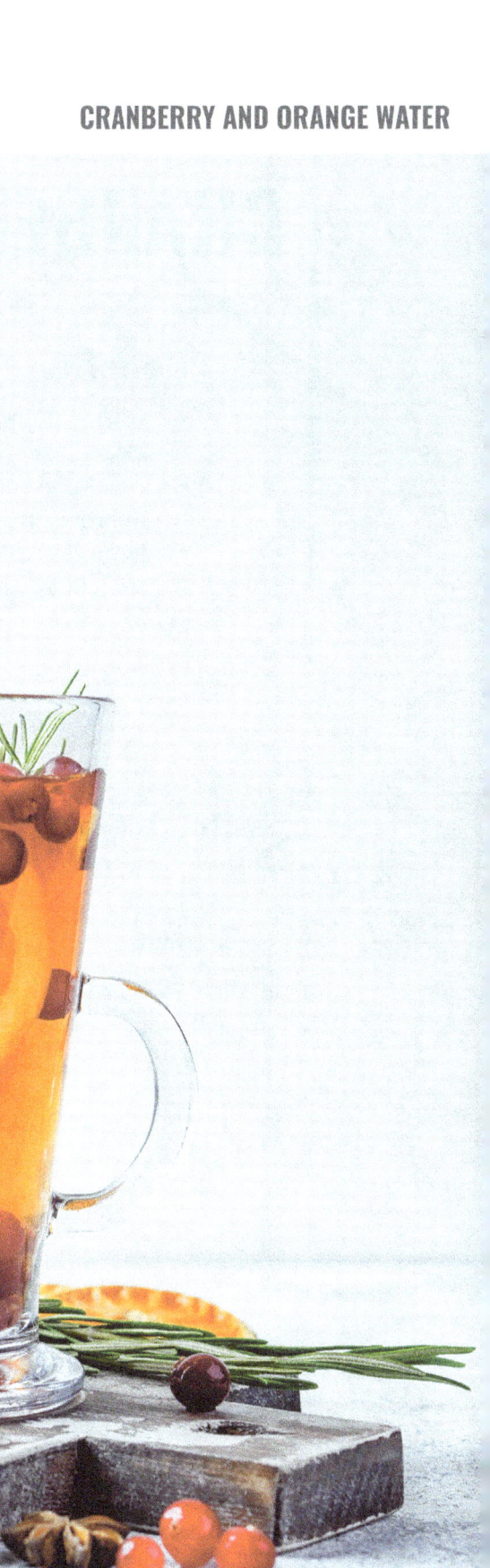

CRANBERRY AND ORANGE WATER

Benefits

- High in antioxidants
- Helps lower risk for UTI
- Helps prevent certain types of cancer
- Improved immune function
- Helps decrease blood pressure
- High in vitamin C

INGREDIENTS

- 2 cups water
- 1 cup fresh cranberries
- 1 small orange

INSTRUCTIONS

1. Slice the orange along with its peel and add it to a pitcher.
2. Add the berries and then mash them with a masher or a spoon.
3. Now add 2 cups of water to fill the pitcher and then let it sit for 2 hours in the refrigerator.
4. Add some ice cubes in the glass and transfer over the ice.

APPLE LIME MINT WATER

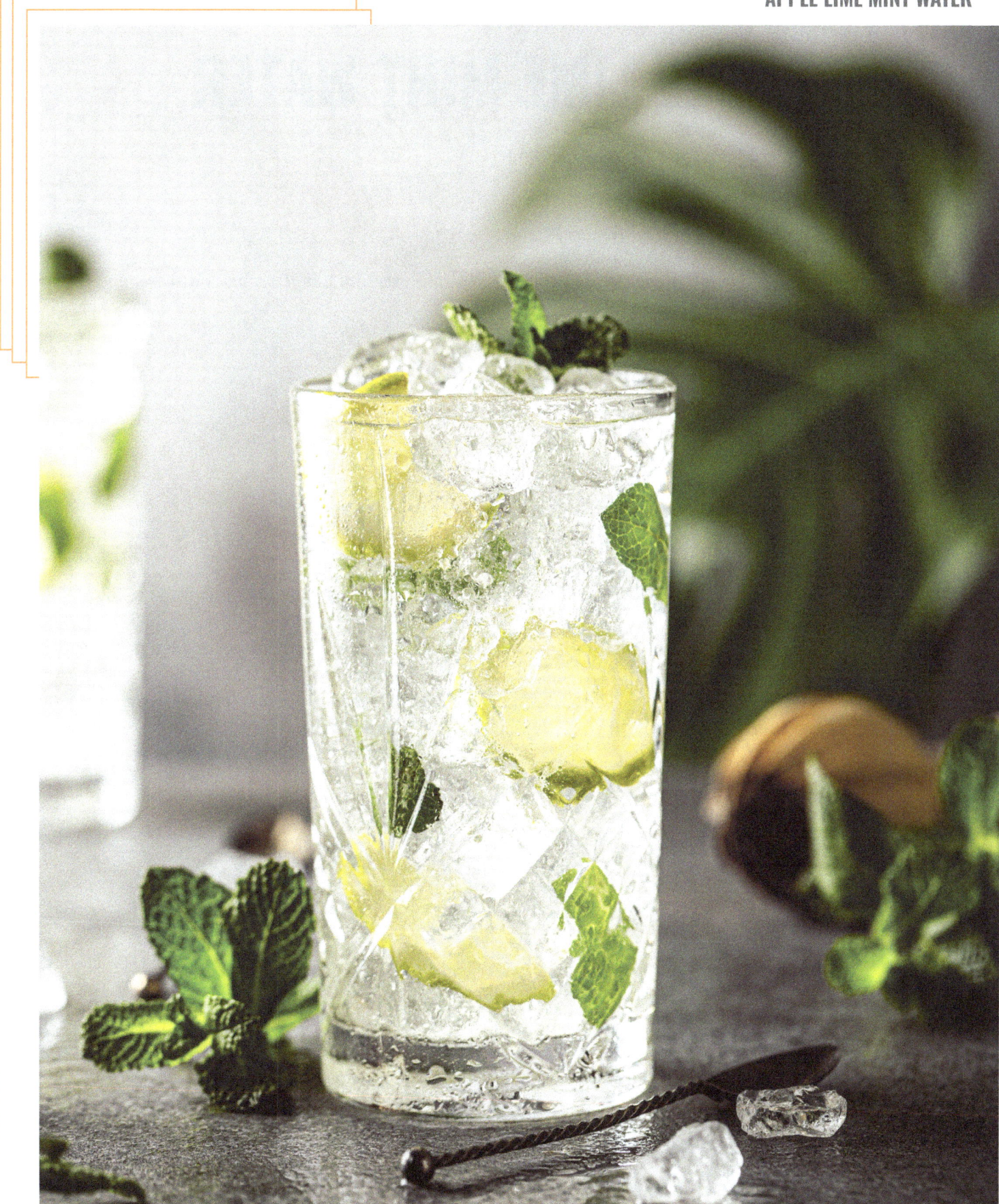

APPLE LIME MINT WATER

Benefits
- High in vitamin C
- Assists with gut health
- Helps reduce risk of stroke, high blood pressure, diabetes, heart disease, obesity, and cancer

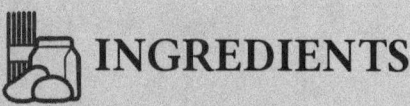 

INGREDIENTS

- 1 Apple
- 4-5 Mint Leaves
- 1 teaspoon date sugar
- 1 teaspoon lemon juice
- A pinch of salt
- 2 cups water

INSTRUCTIONS

1. Grab a blender and blend all the ingredients in it except lemon juice.
2. Prepare a smooth puree, then pass it through a sieve and transfer to a pitcher.
3. Mix lime juice and let it sit in the refrigerator for 2 hours.
4. Serve it chilled and enjoy!

PINEAPPLE AND JALAPENO WATER

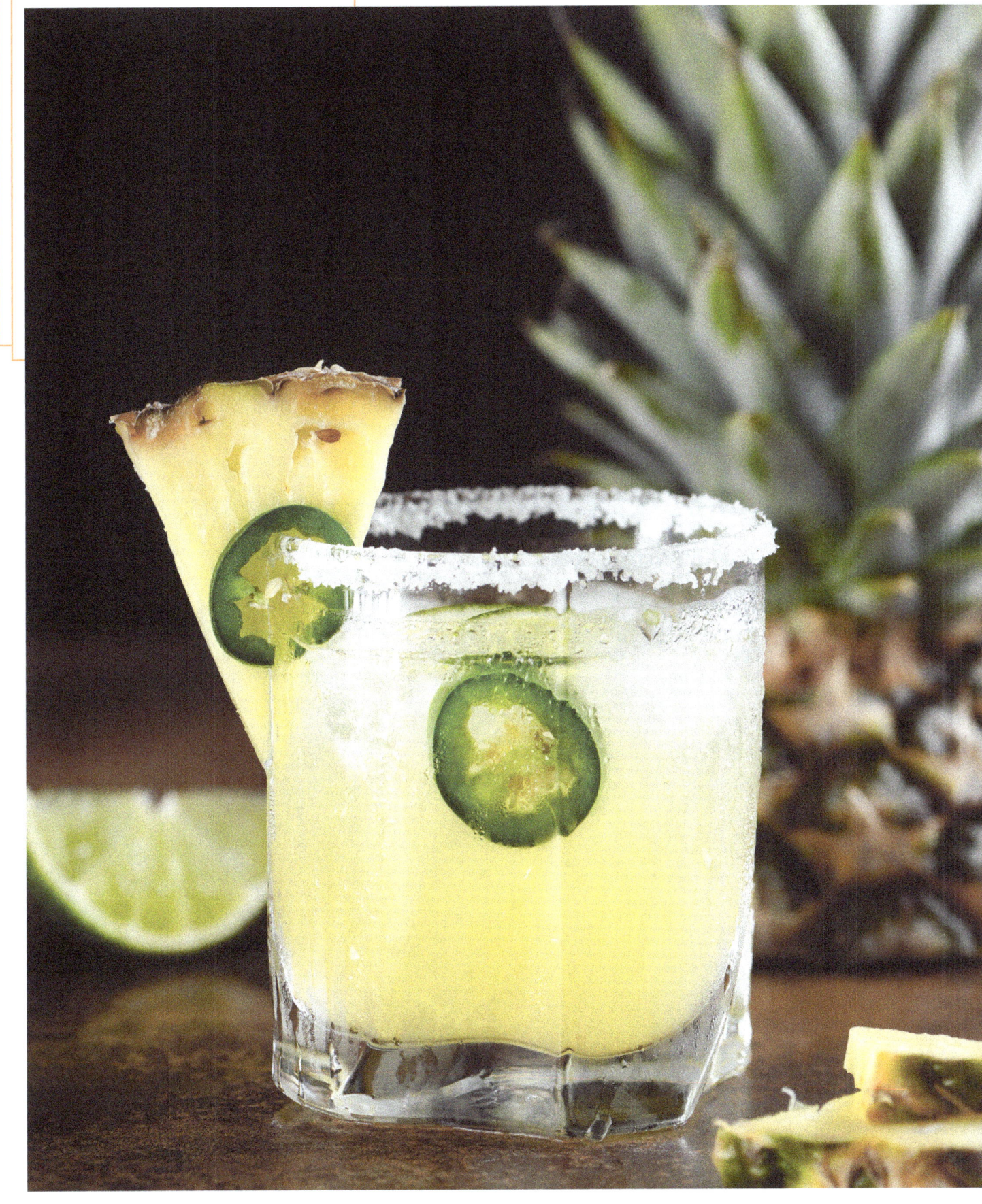

PINEAPPLE AND JALAPENO WATER

Benefits
- Loaded with nutrients and antioxidants
- Enzymes that help with digestion
- Helps reduces the risk of cancer
- Helps boost immune system
- Suppresses inflammation
- Helps ease symptoms of arthritis
- Helps with muscle recovery

INGREDIENTS

- 1/2 cup pineapple
- 1 jalapeno
- Water

INSTRUCTIONS

1. Cut thin slices of pineapple and jalapeno pepper.
2. Put the pineapple and jalapeno pepper slices in a pitcher or a jar.
3. Fill the jar with some water.
4. Refrigerate it for 2-3 hours or leave it overnight to infuse.

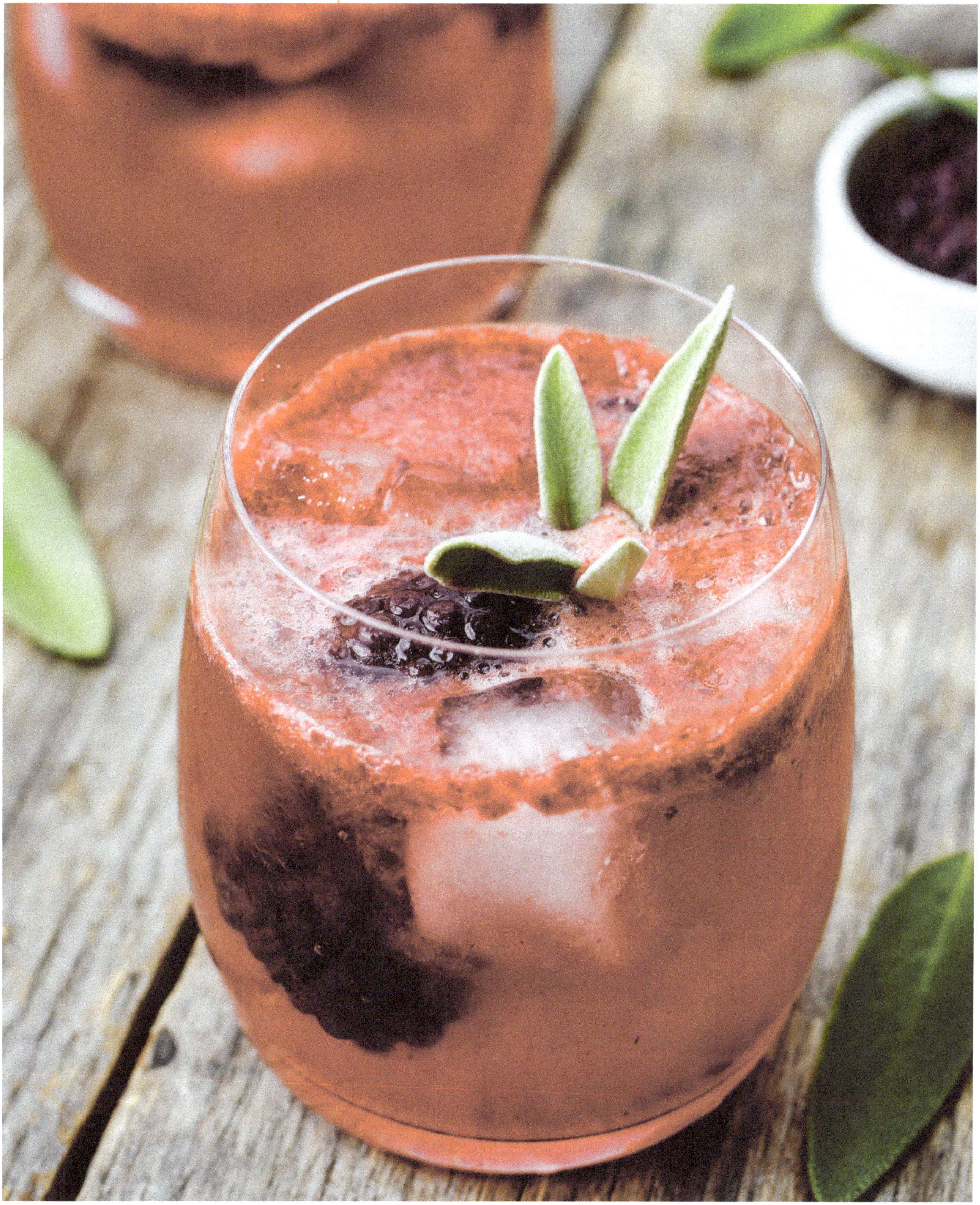

BLACKBERRY ROSEMARY SAGE WATER

BLACKBERRY ROSEMARY SAGE WATER

Benefits

- High in vitamin B6, K, iron, calcium, and manganese
- High in antioxidants
- Helps with oral health
- Helps regulate hormone
- May reduce blood sugar levels
- Supports memory and brain health
- Helps cholesterol
- Helps relieves diarrhea
- Support bone health
- Combats aging skin.
- Helps with hydration

INGREDIENTS

- 2 cups water
- 1 cup fresh blackberries
- 5 springs of rosemary
- 3 fresh sage sprigs
- Ice cubes

INSTRUCTIONS

1. In a jar, combine the blackberries, sage sprigs and rosemary sprigs.
2. Cover the jar and refrigerate it overnight for the best flavors.
3. Strain it before serving and serve with some ice cubes.

CANTALOUPE MINT LEMON WATER

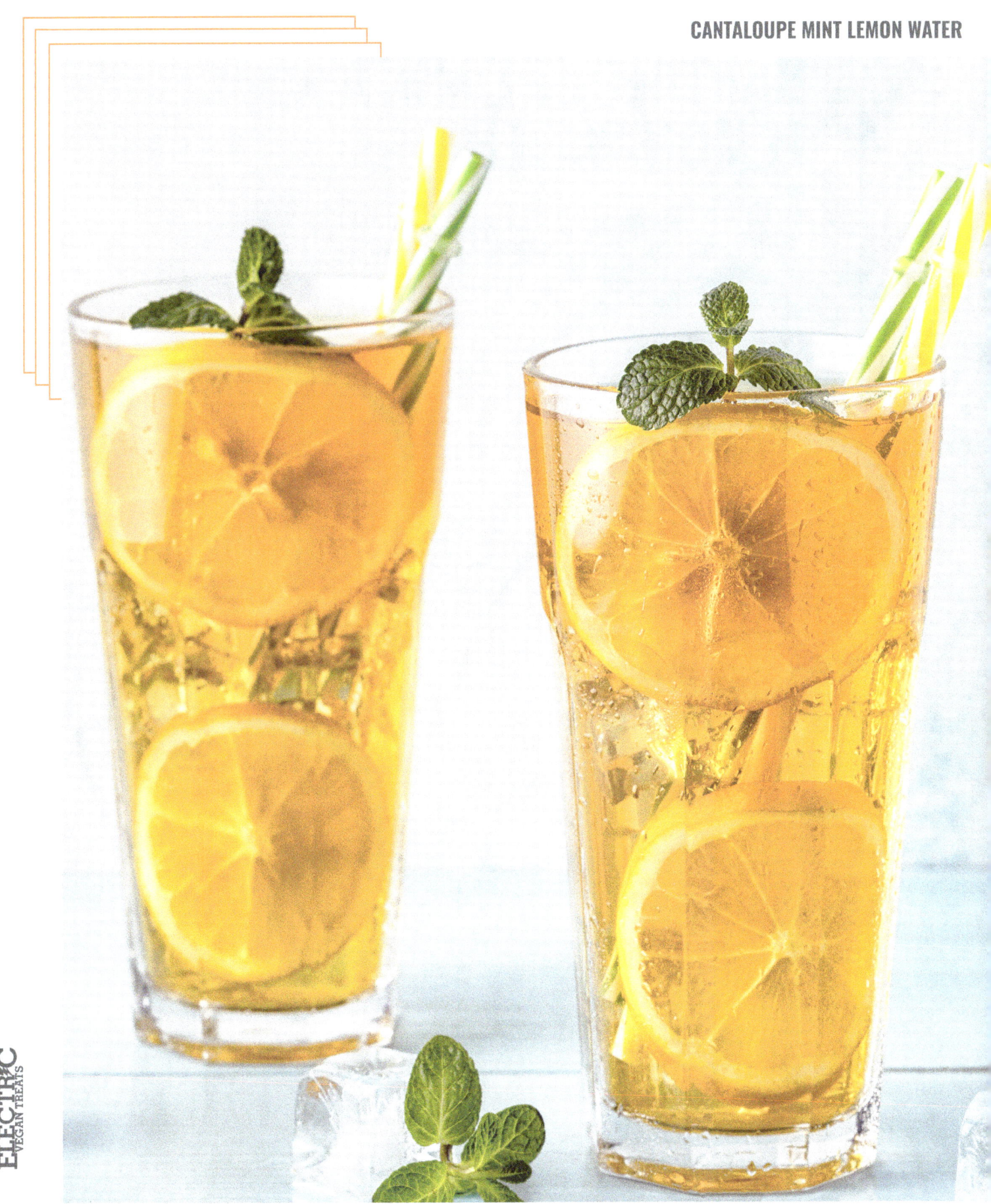

CANTALOUPE MINT LEMON WATER

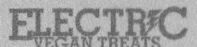

Benefits

- High in vitamin A, C, folate, fiber, and potassium
- Aids in hydration
- Helps detox the body

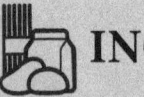 ## INGREDIENTS

 ## INSTRUCTIONS

- 5 fresh mint sprigs
- 1/2 sliced lemon
- 1 cup cubed cantaloupe
- 2 cups of water

1. Grab a pitcher and combine all the ingredients in it.
2. Cover and refrigerate overnight.
3. Serve it chilled with some ice.

PEACHES BASIL WATER

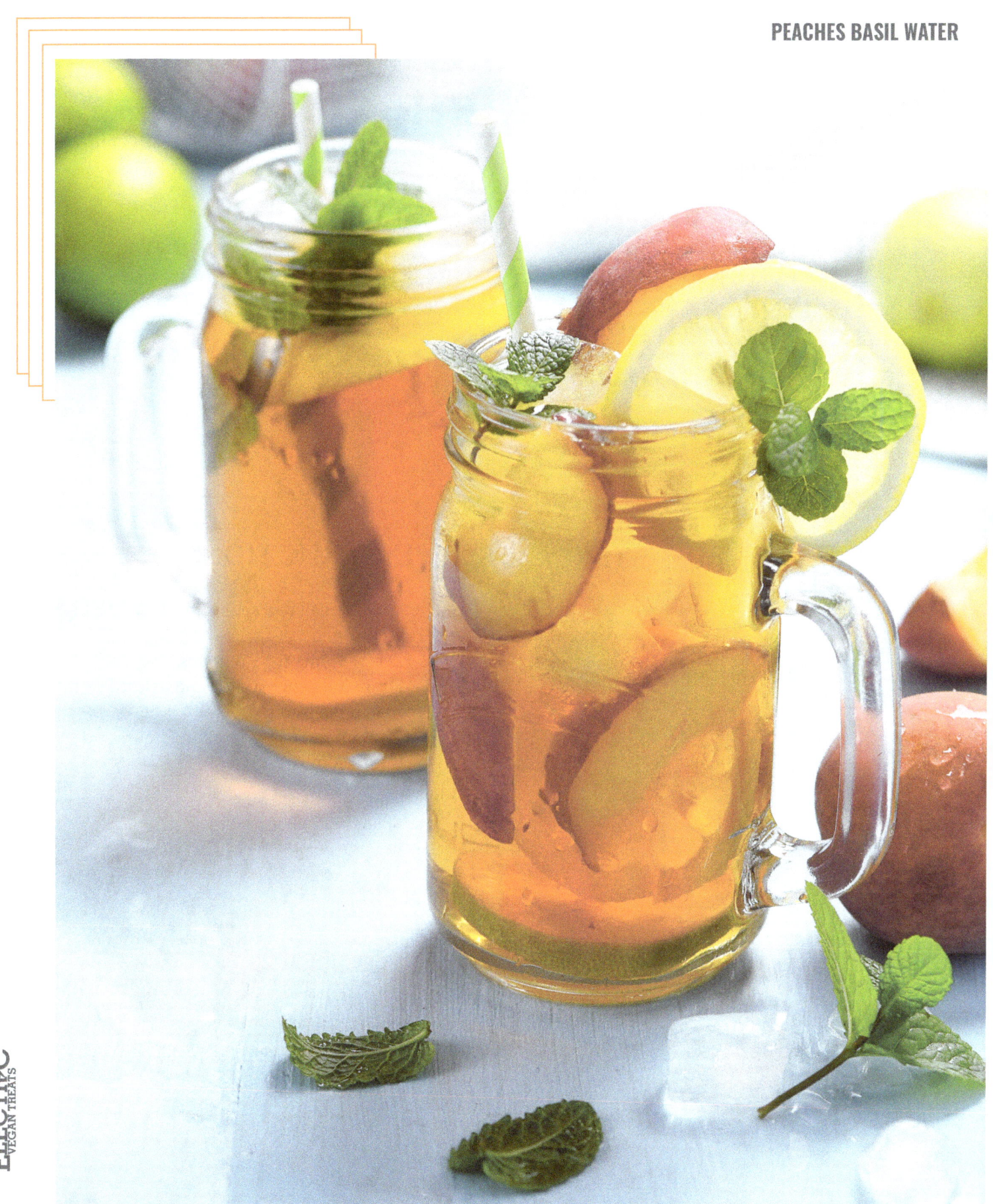

PEACHES AND BASIL WATER

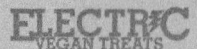

Benefits

- Promotes healing
- Aids in high health
- Aids in digestion
- High in vitamin C
- Keeps bones healthy
- Aids in digestion
- Improves heart health
- Prevents certain types of cancer
- Reduces allergy symptoms
- Protects your skin

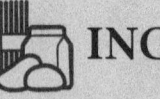

INGREDIENTS

- 1 large sliced fresh peach
- 3-4 tablespoons of basil
- 6 tablespoons of granulated date sugar
- 2 cups of water

INSTRUCTIONS

1. Grab a small saucepan and add all the ingredients in it.
2. Let it simmer for 5 minutes.
3. Strain it through a sieve and discard all the remaining solids.
4. Chill in the refrigerator for 4 hours and serve it with some ice.

CHERRY LIME WATER

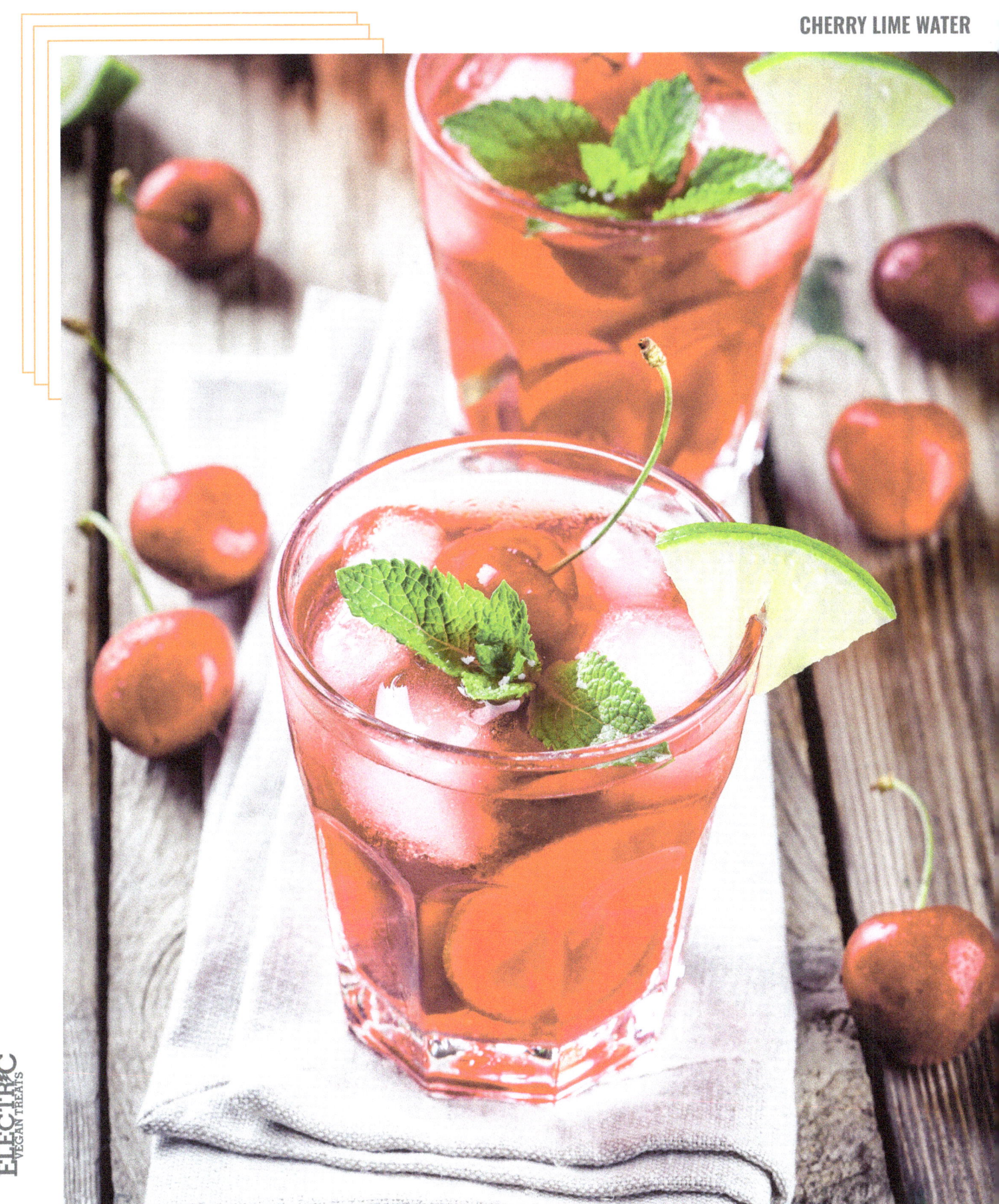

CHERRY LIME WATER

Benefits

- High in Vitamin C, potassium, Cooper, manganese, and fiber
- High in antioxidants
- Anti-inflammatory properties
- Muscle recover
- Benefits heart health
- Improves symptoms of arthritis and gout

INGREDIENTS

- 1/2 cup date sugar
- 2 cups water
- 1/2 cup lime juice
- 1 1/2 cups pitted cherries
- Ice cubes

INSTRUCTIONS

1. Grab a saucepan and combine date sugar and 2 cups of water.
2. Let them boil until the date sugar completely dissolves.
3. Remove from heat and let it cool.
4. Take a blender and pulse the cherries with lime juice.
5. Transfer water date sugar mix in the blender and again give them a good mix.
6. Now add some ice cubes in the blender and pulse them for 2 minutes.
7. Transfer to the serving glass and enjoy the chilled awesomeness!

Electrically Infused Water Recipe Book .

Type of Work:	Text
Registration Number / Date:	TXu002273604 / 2021-08-03
Application Title:	Electrically Infused Water Guide .
Title:	Electrically Infused Water Recipe Book .
Description:	Electronic file (eService)
Copyright Claimant:	Ivana Barnes, 1990- . Address: 11842 Carson Lake Dr W, Jacksonville, FL, 32221, United States.
Date of Creation:	2021
Authorship on Application:	Ivana Barnes, 1990- ; Domicile: United States; Citizenship: United States. Authorship: text.
Pre-existing Material:	photograph(s)
Basis of Claim:	text.
Rights and Permissions:	Ivana Barnes, (904) 760-7032, electricvegantreats@gmail.com
Names:	Barnes, Ivana, 1990-

www.ingramcontent.com/pod-product-compliance
Lightning Source LLC
Chambersburg PA
CBHW081509080526
44589CB00017B/2698